CW00731116

# VOICES *of* HOPE

Inspirational stories of deaf children
listening and speaking,
told by their families

collated by
Estelle Gerrett, LSLS Cert AVT

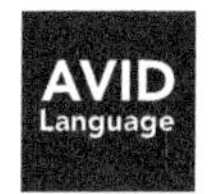

**VOICES OF HOPE**

Published by AVID Language Limited, 3 Cam Drive, Ely CB6 2WH, UK
First published in 2024

**ISBN:**
**Paperback: 978-1-913968-52-6**
**Hardcover: 978-1-913968-54-0**
**eBook: 978-1-913968-64-9**

Collation and editing by Estelle Gerrett
Layout and additional editing by Tanya Saunders for AVID Language Ltd.
Text © Estelle Gerrett 2024
Photographs © Individual Contributors
All rights reserved.

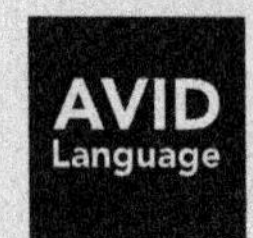


**Inclusive books for families with (and without) hearing loss**

**www.avidlanguage.com**

# Table of Contents

*List of*

# Abbreviations & acronyms

| | |
|---|---|
| ABR | Auditory Brainstem Response (test) |
| ANSD | Auditory Neuropathy Spectrum Disorder |
| AoDC | Adviser on Deaf Children |
| AVT | Auditory Verbal Therapy |
| AVUK | Auditory Verbal UK |
| BSL | British Sign Language |
| CI | Cochlear Implant |
| CMV | Cytomegalovirus |
| EHCP | Education, Health and Care Plan (UK) |
| ENT | Ear, Nose and Throat (department / specialist) |
| FM | FM system/radio aid (an assistive listening device) |
| HDU | High Dependency Unit |
| ICU | Intensive Care Unit |
| IV | Intravenous (line / drip) |
| IP/IEP | Individual (Education) Plan |
| KDEC | Kelston Deaf Education Centre (NZ) |
| MRI | Magnetic Resonance Imaging (scan) |
| NCEA | National Certificate of Educational Achievement |
| NHS | National Health Service (UK) |
| NICU | Neonatal Intensive Care Unit |
| NRT | Neural Response Telemetry (test) |
| ORS | Ongoing Resources Scheme (funding)(NZ) |
| RToD | Resource Teacher of the Deaf |
| SENCO | Special Educational Needs Coordinator |
| TA | Teacher Aide / Teaching Assistant |
| ToD | Teacher of the Deaf |
| NZSL | New Zealand Sign Language |

*This book is dedicated to*
*all the families who have shared*
*their personal stories, experiences*
*and advice in these pages ~*
*with thanks and admiration*
*for their honesty, courage and*
*determination.*

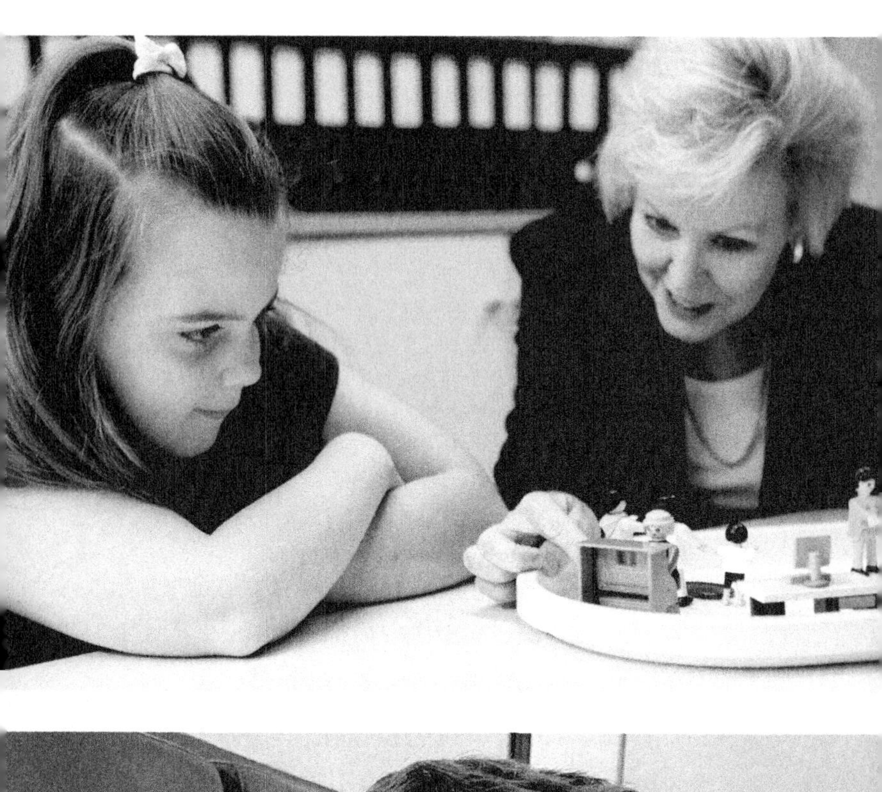

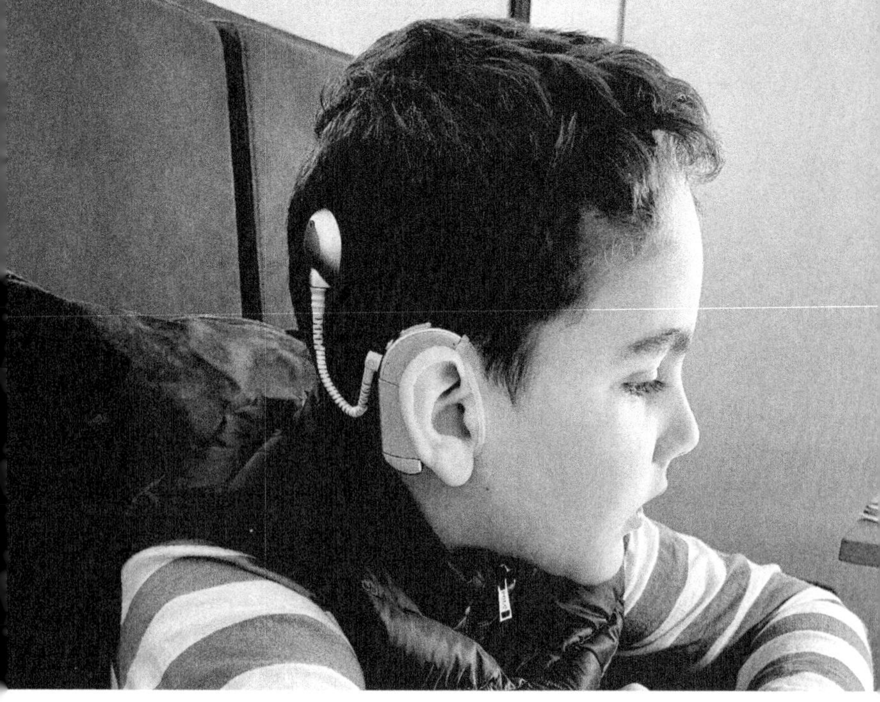

# *Preface*

# Why Auditory Verbal Therapy?

## A HISTORICAL PERSPECTIVE

Auditory Verbal Therapy demands an openness to investigate new scientific evidence, which challenges the established mode of primarily using visual information to help deaf children acquire speech and language. AVT uses strategies in which listening is the primary focus and where parents are the centre of the programme. This is in direct contrast to the earlier prevailing theory that deaf children needed visual information as auditory information was only minimally available. Years ago, this stance was certainly valid and some children with hearing loss did indeed learn to speak when receiving intense speech and language therapy through lip reading and gesture, but now the technology has changed the landscape.

Professor Graeme Clarke and Dr William House's development of the multichannel cochlear implant offered the first device which enabled most children to gain access to all the sounds in the speech spectrum, regardless of the degree of hearing loss. Accordingly, new therapy techniques are needed to match and complement the breakthrough technology.

Professor Clarke said, "The competition from visual brain centers will dominate the auditory brain centres unless we focus on auditory brain access, which is followed by extensive listening experience".

This motivated my and Jacqui Stokes' decisions to pursue the pathway of developing and offering Auditory Verbal Therapy for children in New Zealand and UK respectively. Such statements and convictions became, and still are, the cornerstone declarations to ensure that AVT is available to all children with cochlear implants today.

Today the amount of scientific data supporting AVT has increased significantly. Two generations of children using AVT have become speaking profoundly deaf adults.

The NAL study* has provided the most compelling support yet for the benefits of listening and spoken language input for promoting verbal development in children implanted by three years of age.

**~ Elizabeth Fairgray, Cert AVT**

* The National Acoustics Laboratories study involves:

**I. The study group at the National Acoustic Laboratories:**
Emma van Wanrooy, Patricia van Buynder, Robyn Massie,
Leanne Skinner, Samantha Youn, Alison Jagger,
Nicole Mahler-Thompson, Lauren Burns.

**II. Participating centres, participating investigators:**
Hear and Say Centre: Emma Rushbrooke, Lynda Close
The Shepherd Centre: Maree Doble, Tracey Hopkins
Sydney Cochlear Implant Centre: Kylie Rankine,
Colleen Psarros, Sharan Westcott
Royal Institute for Deaf and Blind Children: Greg Leigh
Strathfield Catholic Centre for Hearing Impaired children
St Gabriel's School for Hearing Impaired children: Lynne Paul
Cochlear implant clinic, Royal Victorian Eye and Ear Hospital
Matilda Rose Early Intervention Centre

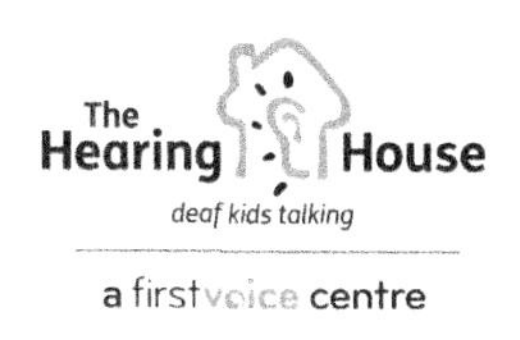


# Introduction to The Hearing House

**www.hearinghouse.co.nz**

Lynne Richards and I get to launch this glorious book that reflects the heart and soul of the original Hearing House. It's a book that talks of passion, determination, and raw courage.

Two of the heroes we sailed with in those early days were mothers of children with hearing loss - skilful teachers, changemakers and leaders of a movement. The first time I met Estelle, who has collated these inspiring stories, it was clear that she was a powerful advocate, a hard worker and had a drive not only to create magic for her son, but for many children with hearing loss. I had been asked to set up a service for children with cochlear implants and had searched the world for the right people to help start the process of achieving the best spoken language results for children with cochlear implants - people with proven skills and knowledge in the field. At the time, cochlear implantation was a controversial subject, as all children in New Zealand schools were taught sign language to communicate.

I soon heard of Judy Simser, a Canadian childhood consultant and teacher who was helping to set up a new centre for children with hearing loss in Taiwan. She was an advocate of Auditory Verbal Therapy and had achieved some outstanding results in North America and Asia. When I contacted Judy, she immediately extended an invitation to visit her in Taiwan (she foolishly said she would make up a bed in her spare room!). The idea was that I would follow her around, observing how she worked with parents, children, therapists and the team of associated professionals – family counsellors, audiologists, surgeons and specialists.

Judy was nothing short of a focused human dynamo. As I watched her work with families, I could see that AVT was a highly effective and empowering methodology to teach children to listen and speak using the technology of cochlear implants. Judy used her vast experience as a mother who had taught her profoundly deaf young son to speak. She had a direct but empathetic approach to teaching parents to teach their children. Her expectations were high, and her results proved that AVT could help profoundly deaf children learn to listen and speak, have a voice, and participate fully in hearing society.

Within months, she was in New Zealand training aspiring therapists like Estelle and wowing a team of visionary professionals who understood that there was a yawning gap to fill.

When you have that sort of momentum, you can't stop. It was intoxicating in those early days. We needed a captain of our clinical ship and history will record all was made possible when we convinced the extraordinarily caring Certified AVT, Lynne Richards, to come to The Hearing House. She helped establish our global reputation as New Zealand's first AVT Centre.

**~ Anne Ackerman, CEO, the original Hearing House**

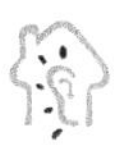

Anne Ackerman as Executive Director of The Hearing House 'inspired all who met her'. She magnificently steered the direction of the Centre with her drive, flair, expertise, and networking skills. She worked tirelessly to fundraise, manage and liaise with all members of The Hearing House family to create a Centre of Excellence. In those early days, there was laughter, pain and tears, but Anne navigated a way to ensure that The Hearing House stood for families with deaf and hard of hearing children - to give them a voice and the very best start in life. The Hearing House would not have galloped along at the pace that it did, without the commitment and dedication of Anne Ackerman.

Children with hearing loss and their parents are very special people and it's unbelievably rewarding to look back on the magic that filled those rooms in the early days. Each family is different and it's easy to remember the first time that children reached age-appropriate language due to the formidable work of their parents and families, all orchestrated by our skilled team of professionals who served them.

We all feel immensely proud and privileged to have been part of The Hearing House in those early foundation years. The Hearing House was founded on love and heart, the generosity of philanthropists who provided the service, dedicated and skilful professionals who shaped the clinical programme and committed families who filled the House with love and laughter as the children learned to listen and speak their minds. This book with its collection of stories reflects this lasting spirit of that early Hearing House.

**~ Lynne Richards, Clinician Lead Cert. AVT**

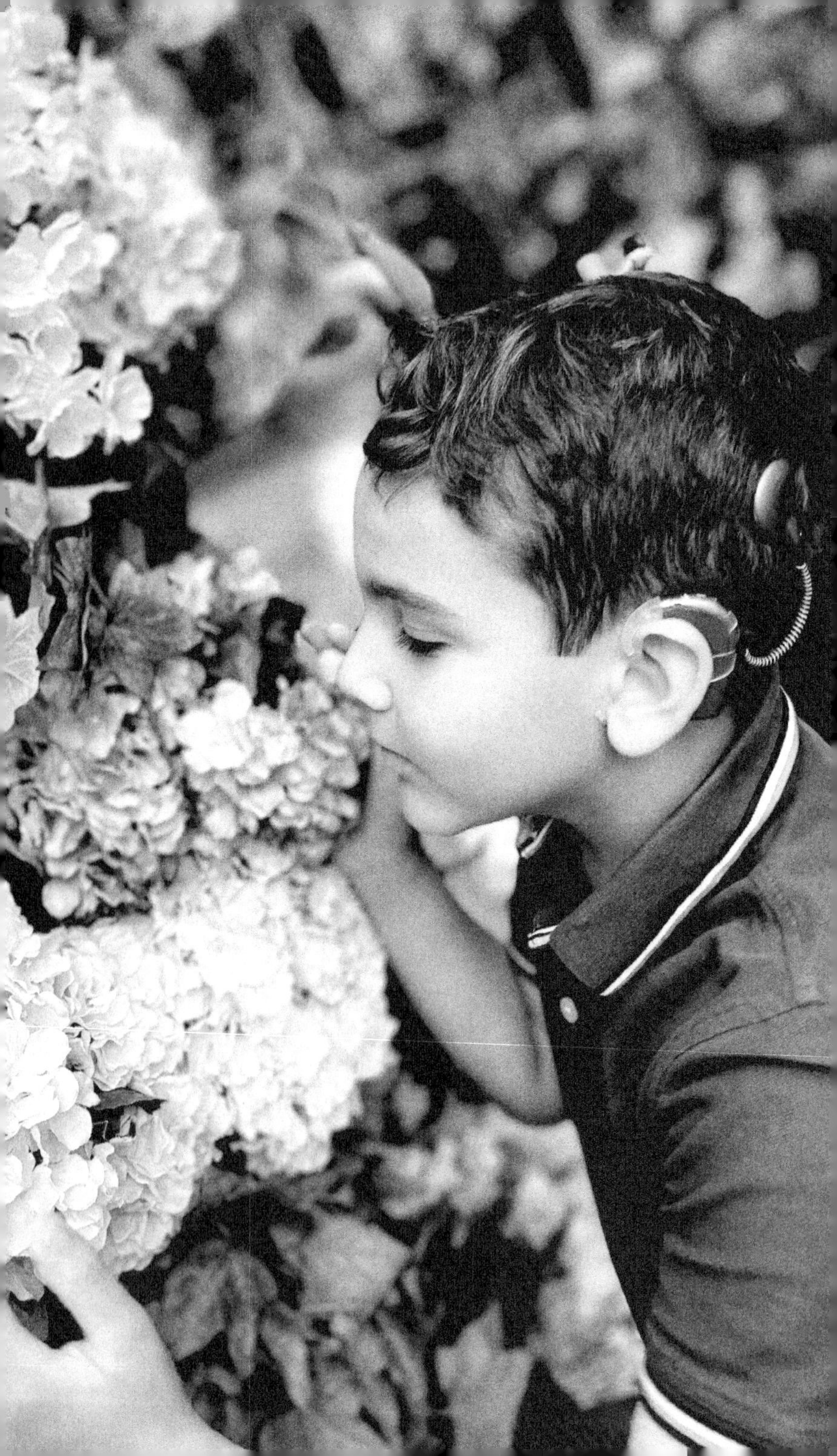

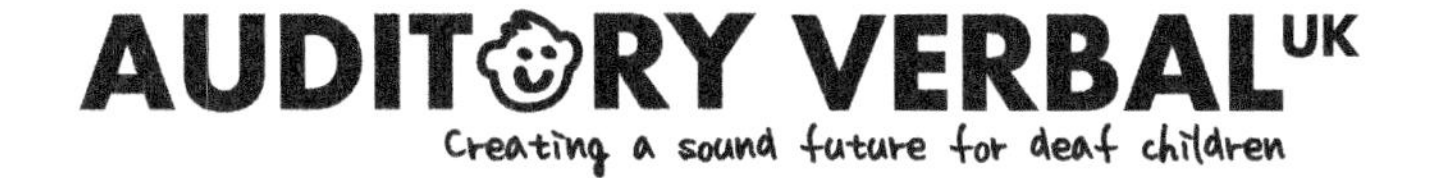


# Introduction to Auditory Verbal UK

**www.avuk.org**

This is an important book for the families of deaf children and the professionals who support them.

It is important because more than 90% of families who have a child who is born deaf or loses their hearing in childhood have no prior experience of hearing loss and deafness. In this book, families share their experiences of what it was like at the start of their journey when they did not know what the future held for their child or what might be possible. Everyone's journey is different and reflects the diversity of deafness, their cultures and the hopes and ambitions that they have for their children.

All children, deaf and hearing, have the right to develop language and communication so that they can achieve their potential in life. Access to the language and communication environment is key to development. For children who are born deaf, especially into hearing families with no experience of deafness, skilled early support is vital if they are to develop language and communication skills. This early and effective support is absolutely crucial whether a family wishes to use spoken language or sign language.

The families in this book talk about their desire for their

children to learn to talk and their experience of Auditory Verbal Therapy.

I first met Estelle Gerrett when I visited The Hearing House in New Zealand and watched her at work, coaching the families of young deaf children using the principles and practice of Auditory Verbal Therapy. Her passion, commitment, professionalism and expertise were so evident. I was delighted that she was able to continue her work at the charity Auditory Verbal UK when she moved to UK in 2017.

Like The Hearing House in New Zealand, Auditory Verbal UK was established to support the families of deaf children in the critical first few years of their lives. AVUK's Founder, Jacqueline Stokes, was the first Auditory Verbal therapist in the UK. She worked tirelessly to demonstrate the listening and talking capabilities of young deaf children and began training practitioners in the UK in the Auditory Verbal approach. Building on her legacy, the charity now provides a family programme, right across the UK, and training in Auditory Verbal practice for speech and language pathologists, educators of the deaf and audiologists around the world, so that every family who wants their child to develop listening and spoken language is able to access a programme close to where they live.

Many people still have low expectations of what deaf children can achieve and many do not know that a profoundly deaf child can learn to talk as well as a hearing child. The stories in this book, as told by the families of young deaf children who have worked with Estelle Gerrett, The Hearing House and Auditory Verbal UK show what is possible and why we can and should have much higher expectations for deaf children and young people around the world.

**~ Anita Grover, CEO, AVUK**

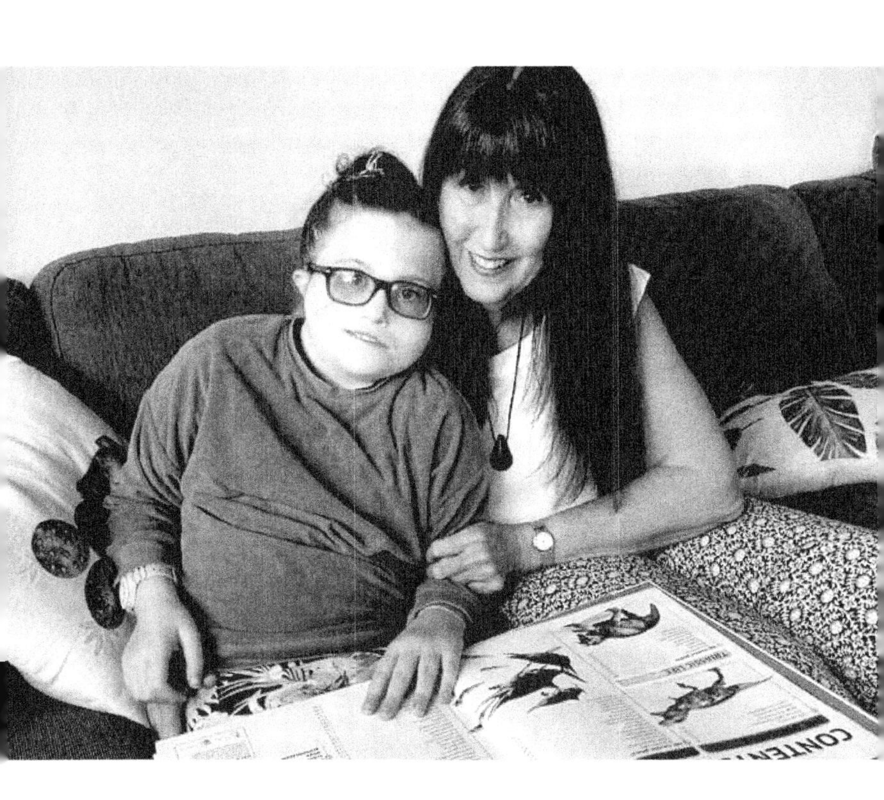

*Hi,*

I have had the privilege of collating this book of stories written by some of the families I have worked with during my career. I have tried to choose a range of families who have faced different diagnoses and different social and cultural challenges, but all have worked to give their children the best spoken language outcome they could achieve through the communication mode of Auditory Verbal Therapy.

My name is Estelle, and I am an Auditory Verbal therapist and mother to three children, now adults. I am passionate about promoting listening and speaking for deaf children to enable them to be full members of a hearing community. My eldest son contracted meningitis at the age of one and was left profoundly deaf. This was a life-changing moment for our family – a moment similar to that faced by all the families in this book.

I embarked on this project because I wanted to have a resource for newly-diagnosed families that was both inspiring and reassuring whilst being open and frank about the challenges faced along the way. These stories represent families from The Hearing House, New Zealand and Auditory Verbal UK in the United Kingdom, as these are the two centres I have worked in.

Most parents who have deaf children are hearing and speaking, and usually crave a spoken outcome for their children. Most have never experienced deafness in their family, and many imagine that the only way to communicate with a deaf person is through sign language. If sign is the family's choice, then it is a full and rich language of its own, but if a spoken language is the family's desire, then learning to listen at an early age will be vital as the foundation for learning to speak.

These thirteen stories present just a small cameo of experiences, which I hope will help readers to understand a little more about Auditory Verbal Therapy and, if they choose to follow this path, to give them hope that their deaf children can be part of the hearing, speaking world.

*Estelle*

**Estelle Gerrett, LSLS Cert AVT, M.Ed HI, B.Ed (Hons) CAES**

*"Extra special children are sent to special people and it will be okay. Your journey will be yours and it will be what it's meant to be."*

~ Sam's Mum

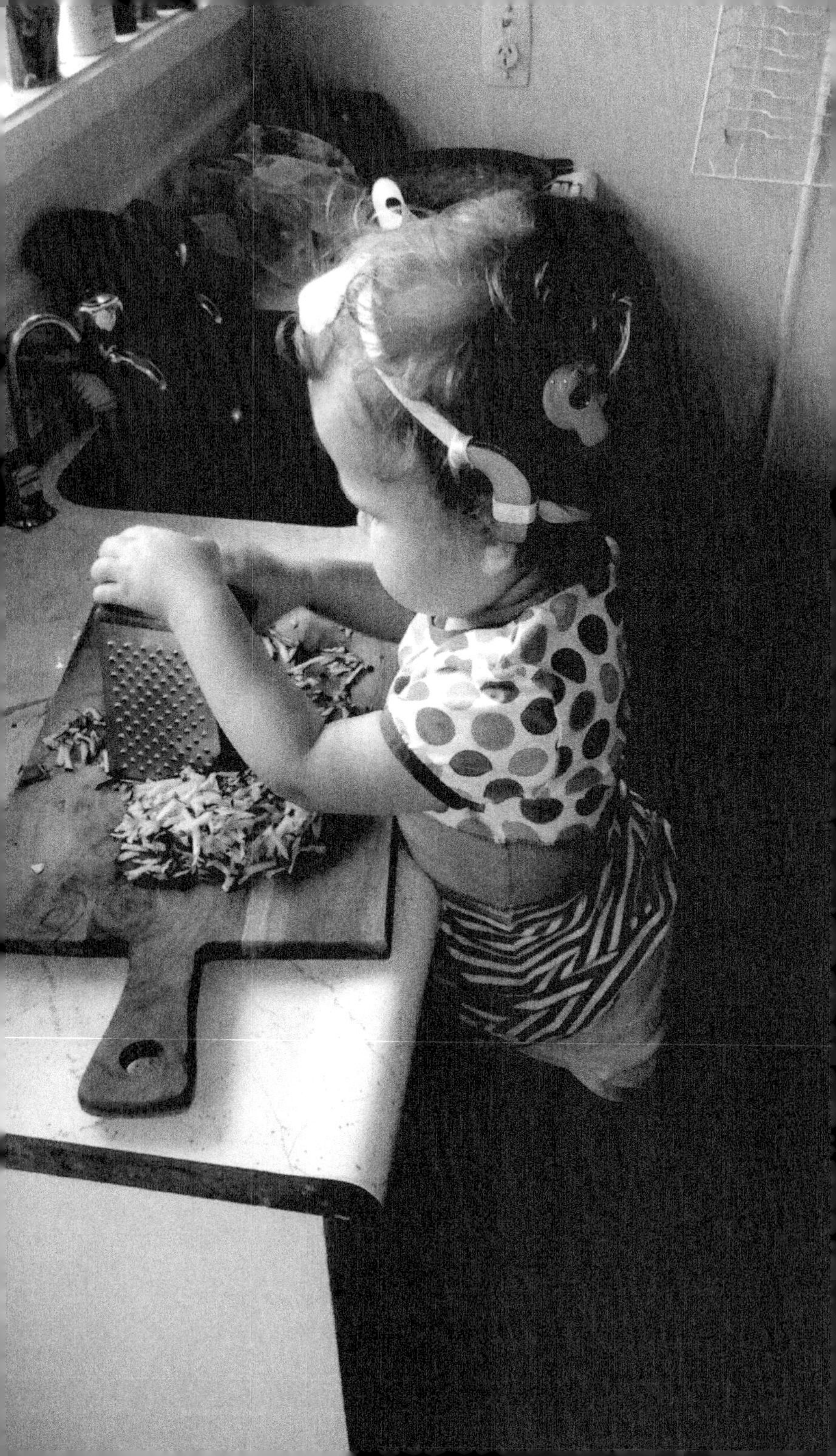

*Lydia's story*

# Our journey to hearing

I sit in a comfy armchair with a sleeping baby on my chest. The room is quiet and calm apart from the occasional beep. The chance to sit quietly is welcome after quite a few weeks of comforting an unsettled colicky baby.

I don't feel the need to ask anything until the last test is finished and my mum asks, "Is it picking up anything?"

The audiologist simply says, "Yes, there is a hearing loss," then leaves the room to get something. This is when I realise my first-born may have something a bit more than a little fluid on the ears...

Rewind six weeks and Lydia was born a few days before full term. A healthy 8lb 12oz baby girl – I was impressed with myself! When she was two days old, while we were recovering at the birth centre, she had a hearing screening test, which she flatlined. We were reassured by the newborn hearing technician that it could just be fluid on the ears from the birth. The test was repeated when she was one week old and again she flatlined. We were told not to worry but referred to Audiology for a proper test. We didn't worry – we had a beautiful newborn baby girl... we had made an ACTUAL BABY!

We stayed with family over Christmas and soon after the break got an appointment with our local audiology service. My husband was back at work, so I asked my mum to come to the appointment – mainly because I hadn't really taken Lydia out by myself yet, not because I was concerned. Before the appointment I had a visit from the Plunket nurse to do the normal well-child checks. She happened to ask if Lydia startled to loud noises. I hadn't seen her do that. We'd been trying to make plenty of noise while she was sleeping. We figured this would teach her to sleep through noise so we wouldn't end up being one of 'those parents' who can't flush the toilet at nap time. It was working! We were feeling kind of pleased with ourselves about that. But this was the first time I had any notion that there might be a problem. By this stage, Lydia was very unsettled and we spent most of this visit talking about her poor sleep, back-arching with feeding and endless crying.

On the day of the audiology appointment, I realised that Lydia was meant to be asleep for one of the tests. I wondered if they were out of their minds and how they expected me to just get this baby to sleep on demand! Mum prayed on her way to my house that Lydia would be settled for the appointment. Lydia was asleep when we got there – they did one test, then she woke up in time for the one she was meant to be awake for. Then the audiologist said she needed to be asleep for the next test... here we go! I did the only thing that seemed to get her to sleep, which was to tie her on me in a Moby Wrap and give her a dummy. I never thought I'd use a dummy but, oh my goodness, they are lifesavers sometimes! I started to do my go-to-sleep sway and within minutes she was asleep. She slept the next two and a half hours while they ran what I now know as a click ABR (auditory brainstem response) test. This is when I got my quiet moment in the comfy chair... until the audiologist returned to the room and showed me the graph of the normal hearing range, then explained the different levels of hearing loss.

"Lydia is in the profoundly deaf range," she said.

Wow! I wasn't expecting that... but I was okay. My mum gave me a hug in case I needed to cry. The audiologist explained she would make the necessary referrals and said Lydia was a strong candidate for cochlear implants. With cochlear implants, she explained, children usually develop normal speech.

We had spent New Year at a friend's house where we had met a woman who had a disability and relied on a wheelchair for mobility. She was an amazing gardener, a beautiful listener and someone who oozed this confidence and groundedness that I so admire. As we left the audiology rooms and made our way to the car, I thought of her. I felt excited by the challenge of raising this beautiful little girl to be confident in herself despite of and because of her 'disability'.

I'm not sure why I felt so calm that day; maybe new mum hormones, maybe the fact that Lydia slept, maybe the lovely audiologist or the reassurance of getting CIs, maybe the challenge (because I do like a challenge) but *'peace that passes all understanding'* comes to mind.

I rang my husband to let him know the news. "She can't hear a bloody thing," I said.

He was a bit shocked but had to push on through as he was a chef and in the middle of his lunch rush (not the greatest timing for a phone call). When he got home, he had time to process and he told me about a dream that had woken him up the night before. It was of his oh-so-lovely grandma, a prayerful Christian lady who had recently passed away. She told him everything was going to be okay. He felt a sense of peace during the dream but didn't know why he had it – now he knew.

A few weeks later and life became very busy (if it wasn't

already busy enough with a new baby). We had visits from our adviser on deaf children, appointments in Auckland, appointments in Hamilton. I felt like I needed my own admin support to keep up with all the appointments and liaise between services. Right before our first trip to Auckland, I finally paid a visit to the after-hours medical centre and got Lydia started on some reflux medication – thankfully she was a whole lot more settled by the next day. We learnt about the cochlear implant assessment process and all the tests and repeat tests that needed to be done prior to surgery.

The next five months are a bit of a blur. I enrolled in some swim lessons for three-month-olds. We went along to check them out. We would sing songs as we moved our babies in the water and then do a countdown 3, 2, 1 before giving them a brief dip underwater as they 'swam' to the instructor. I felt sad for my wee girl that she couldn't hear the cute songs and must have got the biggest fright when she was dipped underwater without hearing the countdown. I did my best to count down on my fingers, but this was challenging when holding her at the same time. I guess without hearing aids our baby didn't 'look deaf', so although I told the swimming instructor, things were done much the same as for the other babies without many extra visual cues.

A couple of general anaesthetics and lots of tests later, Lydia had her cochlear implant surgery at six months old. We were one of the lucky ones to have them offered so early. On the day of the operation, I woke early to breastfeed her before she had to be nil by mouth. I was worried that she would want feeding during the time before surgery, which was against the pre-surgical protocols. We arrived at the Gillies Hospital and were shown to our room. Our Auditory Verbal therapist, Estelle, met us there and talked us through what was going to happen. We also met with the surgeon and anaesthetist. We watched the medical staff dose Lydia with Pamol etc. and then I accompanied her into the theatre while she was put under anaesthetic.

Thankfully, we had planned some activities to do while Lydia was in surgery. A walk up one-tree hill and brunch at a café; we reassured ourselves that Lydia was being cared for by very expensive babysitters... who happened to be doing surgery on her head. In hindsight, we could have planned a few more activities as the surgery took quite a while. For me, the anaesthesia was the scary part and a six-hour surgery felt like a long time for our baby to be under. We had heaps of friends praying for Lydia, which meant a lot to us during that time.

As Lydia came around from the anaesthetic, we settled into our room at Gillies and were super grateful to have time to rest and a nice meal. Lyds was very sleepy overnight but a lot better the next day when they x-rayed her head to check the CI was in place. Then, we headed home.

Just two weeks later, we were back up to Auckland for switch-on. It was super exciting to see our baby girl turn to each new beep. I remember walking through autumn leaves afterwards and the awe of knowing our daughter could be hearing the rustling of leaves for the very first time. It was a beautiful moment. Although, when we look back on the switch-on video now, we're reminded of how exhausted we were from those first, very full-on six and a half months.

The next year we continued to have regular appointments for Auditory Verbal therapy and audiology. We learnt many songs to sing with our girl like, "*I'm a little fish - swish, swish, swish. I swim in water - swish, swish, swish*", something I don't think I would have done as much of without this support. I guess after six and a half months of having a baby who didn't respond to sound, it didn't come naturally.

There was a really challenging stage at around eight months when Lyds realised she could pull her Hearing Henry headband (and 'ears') off. We were warned that she might do it every five minutes – it felt like every two! I ended up dressing her in a little red balaclava as it was the only thing she didn't seem to be able to pull off. I've since found some really pretty bonnets on Etsy... but you do your best with the knowledge you have at the time. We pushed through that exhausting phase and I'm glad we did because it was in the next few months that we really saw her begin to respond to and enjoy sound.

I learnt to build on Lydia's language by giving back a little bit more than she gave to us. She'd give a sound, we'd give a word. She'd give a word - "eyes" was the first - we'd give her two: "Mummy's eyes". She'd give a phrase, we'd give a sentence.

While we taught Lydia to listen and speak, we also chose to learn New Zealand Sign Language as a family with some help from some very lovely Deaf adults. We were keen to give her as much access to communication as we could and used this at bath time and bedtime once her 'ears' were off. Around her first birthday she began to sign "food", then "more food", and not long after that began to speak.

There were times the hearing and sign worked together. She would hear a helicopter fly above the house and sign "helicopter". A bit later on we heard her babbling a very long sentence about a "coptapopta" and worked out that she was probably telling us about a helicopter.

When Lydia was around eighteen months old, the stress of the past year and a half caught up with us and I struggled with anxiety. I learnt not to underestimate the benefits of a good night's sleep, time to oneself, exercise and just sitting outside listening to the birds.

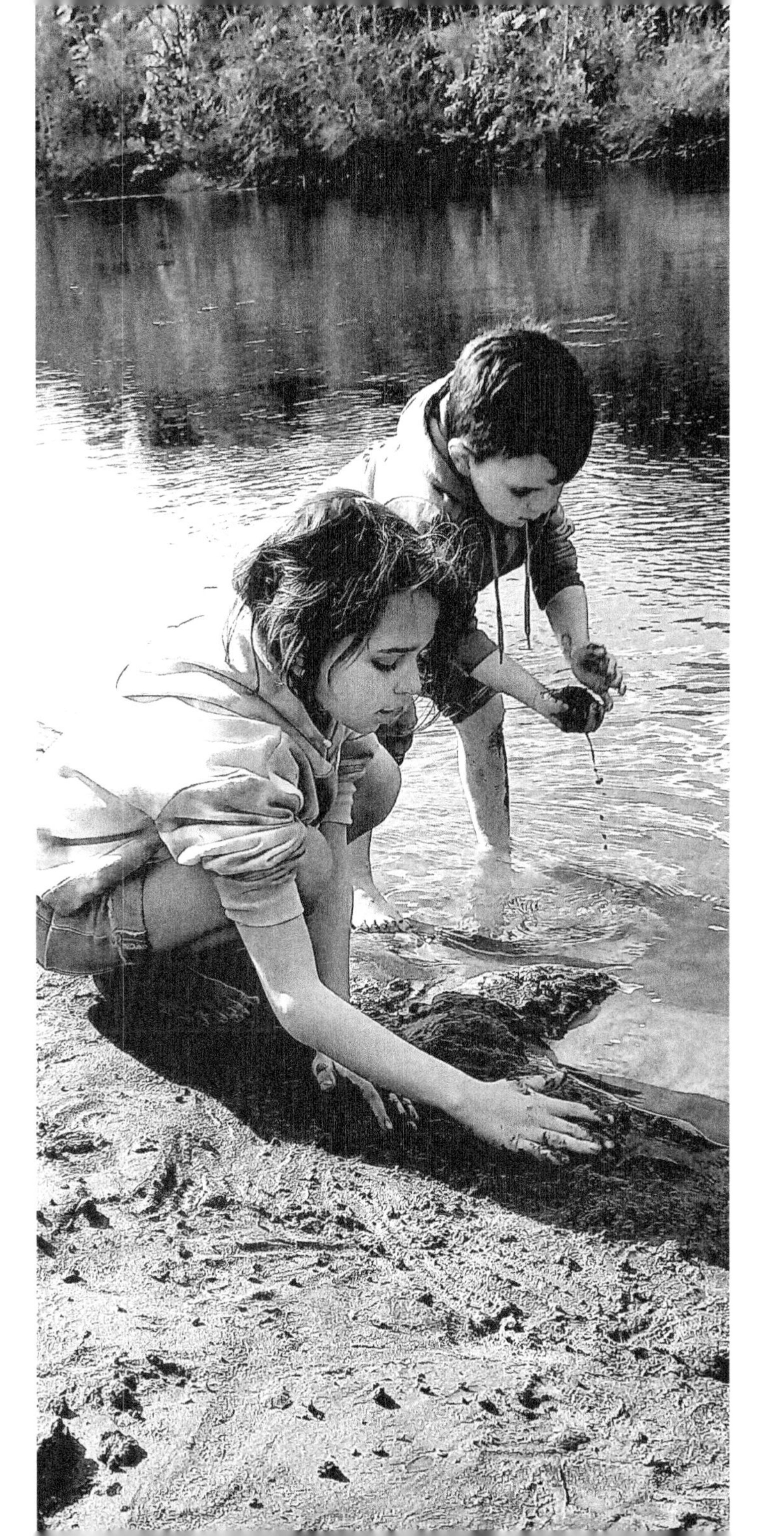

I went back to work part time and we continued Auditory Verbal Therapy, although less frequently. As Lydia has learnt language at a much faster pace than we could, English has become her preferred language; after all, it is what we are fluent in.

When Lydia was about two, I remember playing on repeat a song from daycare that Lydia loved, which went *"savalivali means go for a walk, tautalatala means too much talk"*. It was such a delight to see our girl enjoying music and language. She's always been a kid who is determined to learn and to communicate. At one point, she tried to climb the back fence telling us that she was on her way to the moon.

Lydia's dad remembers some challenging parenting moments when Lydia would take her 'ears' off when she didn't want to stop her play. She would hide her 'ears' and refuse to look up so that she didn't have to be interrupted.

Fast forward a few years and she is now a tenacious seven-year-old who loves reading and doesn't seem to be short of friends. It took her a while to build up courage to put her head under the water at swim lessons but she got there and wears an aqua ear for swimming now. She has her moments when she needs time to herself and some peace and quiet but for the most part is a happy, confident kid with amazing vocabulary.

We are super grateful for all the support we have received along our journey from our audiologist, AODC, Auditory Verbal therapists, The Hearing House, First Signs programme, family, friends, church whanau and school. It's been an amazing journey and we're still travelling it.

*Onna's story*

# Choosing speech

Bedtime story completed, twins kissed goodnight and wrapped up in bed. One of them – the one who is deaf – reaches out her little hand to me and says, "Mummy, please don't go. I want to talk. I want to talk all night. I love talking."

My Mummy-heart just about burst in that moment. It's hard to explain everything which that brief instant represented in our family life: the long accumulation of love, fear, determination, hope, exhaustion, perseverance, doubt, belief, obstacles, milestones, setbacks, progress, questions, answers that all seemed contained within those few simple words from our daughter. Overwhelmingly, they validated for me the choices her father and I had made – had had to make – on her behalf when she was first diagnosed as profoundly deaf, shortly before her third birthday.

We were living in Kenya at the time, but our story started in New York City, where Onna and Sala had surprised us with their unexpectedly early arrival into the world – they were born at 28 weeks and spent over sixty days in the neonatal intensive care unit. Some few months later, we were able to fly home to Kenya with them. They had both passed their newborn hearing screening before being discharged from the NICU so, two years down the line when we were told not to worry about Onna's hearing, we made the mistake of doing exactly that. Because she had passed her newborn

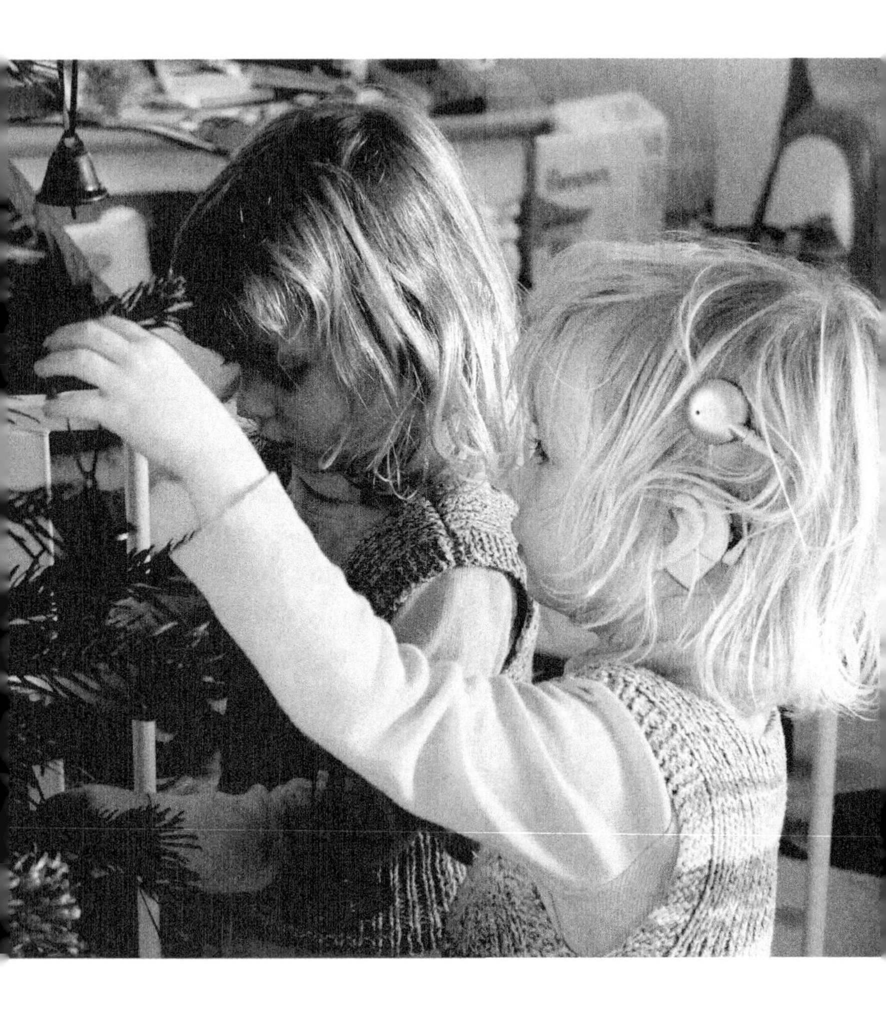

screening, we believed the glue ear diagnosis must be right. We had no reason to doubt the diagnosis until, a few months later, we were on holiday in UK and decided to seek a second opinion, just for safety. That's when our lives were turned upside down.

We discovered the truth: Onna was deaf. She had severe-profound sensorineural hearing loss and auditory neuropathy spectrum disorder (ANSD) in both ears. Her only chance of ever learning to listen and speak was to get bilateral cochlear implants and undergo intensive speech and language therapy.

And yet, despite the bombshell that had landed in our midst, we did not hesitate – the decision came swiftly and naturally to us (in this I think we were fortunate, because procrastination may have muddied the waters for us). Nothing would stand in our way - we would change our lives completely in order to provide both our daughters with the best life chances possible – and there was no time to lose. So, having arrived in England for what we thought would be just a ten-day visit with family, the twins and I suddenly found ourselves house-hunting, while Ian went back to Kenya to close down our entire former life.

Onna had bilateral cochlear implant surgery just as she was turning three years old. At that point she was completely nonverbal. As for her father and me, we had been thrown into a completely new world about which we knew absolutely nothing, but our initial research told us one vital thing: early intervention is key when teaching a deaf child to listen and speak. We learned (to our dismay) that the first three years of a child's life are critical for the development of language, but you still have a pretty good window of opportunity until they are five. After that, things get much tougher – not impossible, but tougher and slower. Onna, aged three and only just having gained access to sound through her cochlear implants, was classed as a 'neurological emergency'. We had to start stimulating her auditory brain as soon as possible. Ian and I had no idea of the scale or nature of the task ahead, nor precisely what it would entail, but we knew we would do whatever was necessary to help Onna develop speech and language and all the cognitive, emotional and social skills that go alongside. Our ultimate goal and constant guide through the many decisions which faced us in those early days was this: We wanted Onna to be able to access the same opportunities in life as her typically-hearing twin sister, Sala.

It goes without saying that we respect every family's right to choose their own communication approach for their deaf children. All parents make life-defining choices for their young children at various points throughout their childhood, and many of these choices are not easy. When it comes to choosing a communication approach for your deaf child(ren), I don't believe there is a 'one size fits all' solution. Everyone has different circumstances and different values, and the choice each family makes is a very personal decision and not for others to judge.

While wishing to give Onna the same chances in life as her sister, we chose to pursue a listening and spoken language approach for many additional reasons too. We believe immersion in a fluent language environment is the best way to learn any language. With the best will in the world, Ian, Sala and I were not going to become fluent in British Sign Language quickly enough to give Onna the intensive language support she needed straight away, delaying even further her access to a fluent language environment. With spoken English, we could provide this straight away – spoken English was all around us at home and everywhere we went in our everyday life.

We also believe that being able to listen and speak will open up many more life choices for Onna in the end, not to mention a much wider social, family and friendship circle. Realistically, even if her father, sister and I learnt BSL, if Onna only communicated in sign language, how many others would do so fluently enough to build full, meaningful relationships with her? How many education and employment opportunities would be open to her without hearing and speech? We had to be pragmatic and realistic about our choices for her. Like it or not, we live in a world driven by spoken and written communication. It's a hard reality to face as the parents of a newly-diagnosed deaf child, but it was our responsibility to face it and make the choices for Onna, which we felt would give her an equal chance in life. *Let's do the hard work early on so that her life is easier later on,* we thought.

We would never dissuade Onna from learning sign language as a second (third or fourth) language, if she ever wanted to. (Indeed I frequently talk to her about this now and tell her that if she ever wants to learn BSL, I will learn alongside her. She's not keen at the moment, but may change her mind in future.) But, to begin with, especially as she had already missed so much time due to her late diagnosis, we felt it better to concentrate all our efforts on a single mode of communication.

Having decided to focus one hundred percent on spoken language, we chose to enrol Onna in the Auditory Verbal therapy programme run by Auditory Verbal UK because we liked their aspirational, diagnostic-led approach, which mirrored Ian's and my attitude to life in general: reach for the stars while keeping your feet firmly grounded in reality. We knew Onna was going to have to play catch-up and work very hard, as she had missed out on three years of hearing, which put her a long way behind her peers in speech and language. She also had ANSD to deal with, so there was an awful lot for her brain to figure out before she could start putting it together and make sense of it all. Later, we discovered that both her implants were failing, so she had been contending with that too. It's no wonder, perhaps, that things moved so slowly to begin with. Onna worked hard, we worked hard, progress was coming but slowly, slowly. At times, we know that some people questioned whether we were making the right decision to pursue a listening and spoken language approach with her, yet we kept seeing small but definite indicators of progress, especially at home, even if she would not always 'perform on cue' when at nursery or during her therapy sessions. These glints of progress gave us hope and helped us to hold our nerve, which wasn't always easy. We continued to trust our gut-feeling that Onna would get there in the end – she would do it at her own speed, but she would get there. And then, after about eighteen to twenty months of AVT, Onna suddenly seemed to turn a corner, and her progress since then has been exponential.

When she was six years old, she underwent revision surgery to replace both her failing implants. She sailed through the surgery and recovery much more smoothly than I thought possible, and the new implants immediately started working wonders for her.

Onna has always faced her challenges with such determination, courage and joy. She is a happy child and this, above all, is our yardstick. If she were miserable or frustrated, we would question the choices we have made and are still making for her. She is now ten years old, is a complete chatterbox and has age-appropriate reading skills (she is a bookworm). She loves music, gymnastics, tennis, swimming and riding her bike, is forming strong friendships and, supported by wonderfully dedicated teaching assistants, attends mainstream school alongside her twin sister. Her grammar is still a little patchy at times, but her functional ability to communicate is excellent. Onna manages to keep up with her schoolwork, proving how resilient she is - she is finding her own special way to make the world work for her, despite the tricky path that fate has laid before her. She still has to work very, very hard but her progress now is remarkable – her strides forward take our breath away. Subjects like maths, which (ironically) require such attention to the subtlety of language, have been difficult for her but have failed to dampen her enthusiasm for learning. She and her sister, Sala, with her equally sparkling personality and many talents, make us proud and grateful every single day. Both girls, in traveling this road together, have learned many life skills early on that will stand them in good stead when they reach adulthood. It's a hard world out there, not always fair or even logical and there's a lot to be said for being able to find a way through, no matter which obstacles lie in your path, never giving up, seeing the positives instead of only the negatives in any given situation, and being able to retain a sense of humour through it all. One of the things which has been so wonderful to observe as Onna's language has developed is her glorious sense of humour transitioning from purely physical expression to verbal expression. As a family, we do laugh a lot.

If I had the space here, there are many seminal moments I could share with you from our journey so far, and I'm sure many of you will recognise them from your own journeys – the first time your child said "Mummy" or "Daddy" or, before that, the first time they turned to the sound of their name being called. These may seem like small steps for some people but are huge strides in our world.

And yet, when I think about the mountain Onna has had to climb and is still climbing, it's hard not to think of the 'what ifs'. *What if we had taken her to see a specialist sooner? What if she had got her cochlear implants two years earlier? How much easier would it have been for her?* These are questions which can drive you crazy. We are where we are. But whenever the parents of newly-diagnosed, profoundly deaf babies ask me for my opinion as to whether they should get cochlear implants for their babies straight away or wait and see if things improve, or even whether they should wait until their children are old enough to make the decision for themselves, my answer is always the same: if you want your child to learn to speak, do it now and start therapy to stimulate their auditory brain as soon as possible. Do it as soon as you can because the longer you leave it, the harder it is for your child.

And my second piece of advice is this: as a parent, be prepared to immerse yourself in your child's hearing loss journey, for this offers your child the best chance of success. There is no better guide, no stronger advocate, no greater champion of your child than you. This was another thing that attracted us to AVT: it puts parents in the driving seat. Your Auditory Verbal therapist will continue to check in with your child to monitor their progress and set appropriate goals, but above all they will train you as the parent to guide and inspire your child along their listening and spoken language journey. No one has a greater incentive to see their child succeed than the parents, no one spends more time with their child when they are young, and no one knows their child as well, so parents are ideally placed to drive their child's progress. AVT constitutes more than just a schedule of therapy sessions; it becomes a lifestyle. For it to work best, it needs to be integrated seamlessly into every aspect of family life. This is not as hard as it sounds – your therapist guides you every step of the way and very soon it becomes second nature.

We have also seen wider benefits, which have indirectly (or perhaps directly) derived from our AVT journey. I believe it made learning to read (which can be tricky for deaf children) easier for Onna because she had learned how to listen carefully and focus on specific sounds, which helped her to grasp phonics. And because AVT is a 'whole world' approach, it does so much more than just focus on the mechanics of listening and speech, but supports a child to develop self-confidence, theory of mind and emotional intelligence. These qualities are so important for social integration, which can be a struggle for some deaf children. From my experience with my two children, I have seen that interpersonal skills tend to develop naturally over the course of childhood in parallel with language but in the case of a child who is deaf, may need to be taught more purposefully.

Raising a deaf child to listen and speak requires a team effort, involving family, friends and professionals from many different disciplines. To be most effective, one parent needs to become the *de facto* 'team leader'. This can feel daunting, especially in the face of so many different options. AVT, with its strong parent-coaching component gave me the skills, knowledge and confidence in my own instincts as a parent to build this team around Onna, to become her strongest advocate, able to engage confidently and constructively with the professionals working with her, and to leverage the maximum support available within the bounds of the choices we had made for her. It was vital for this diverse team to stay 'on the same page' and pull in the same direction, even in the face of occasional disagreements regarding our choice of therapy and communication approach, educational setting and aspirations for the future.

Onna left the AVUK programme many years ago now, but I still use Auditory Verbal strategies every single day at home, both with Onna and Sala. Onna has continued to have a strong support network around her, including dedicated hearing loss professionals (particularly her outstanding teacher of the deaf and audiology team), as well as her fabulous school, which has always provided such a nurturing, inclusive and motivating environment for her. When it comes to the people who have worked with Onna in the past, and those who continue to work with her and our family, I feel like we have won the lottery. It is thanks to all of them that Onna is now making such fantastic progress – combined with her miracle technology, her own hard work, her twin sister's absolute dedication and all the family's wholehearted commitment - but I still trace back the root of her current progress to the foundation built by AVT, which six years ago opened a doorway in Onna's auditory mind and taught her first and foremost to listen, as the basis for later learning to speak. This is a long road we're on, it's a hard road and it can be bumpy – and we still have quite a way to go – but now that we are on it, I wouldn't change it for the world.

I started these musings with one of many anecdotes that stand out from this remarkable journey we are on, as Onna forges her way into the hearing and speaking world. So now, to end, I leave you with another. Again, it's bedtime, again I'm leaning in to kiss our two beautiful daughters goodnight, and Onna stretches up her little arms to me.

"I love you," she says (for the very first time in her life) and then she rolls over to Sala, her twin sister, and says, "I love you, too."

Oh, my heart! Cue tears. Enough said.

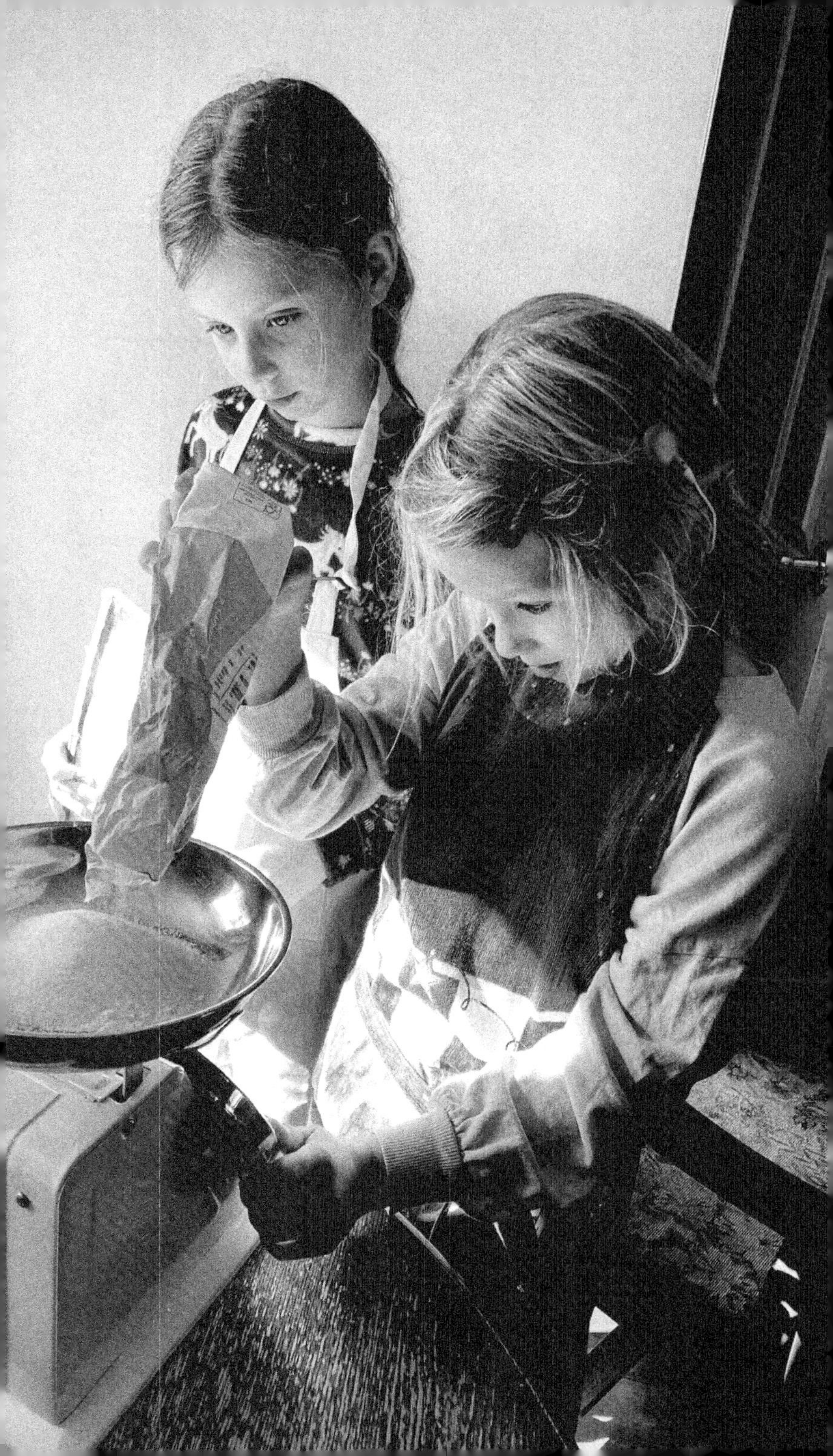

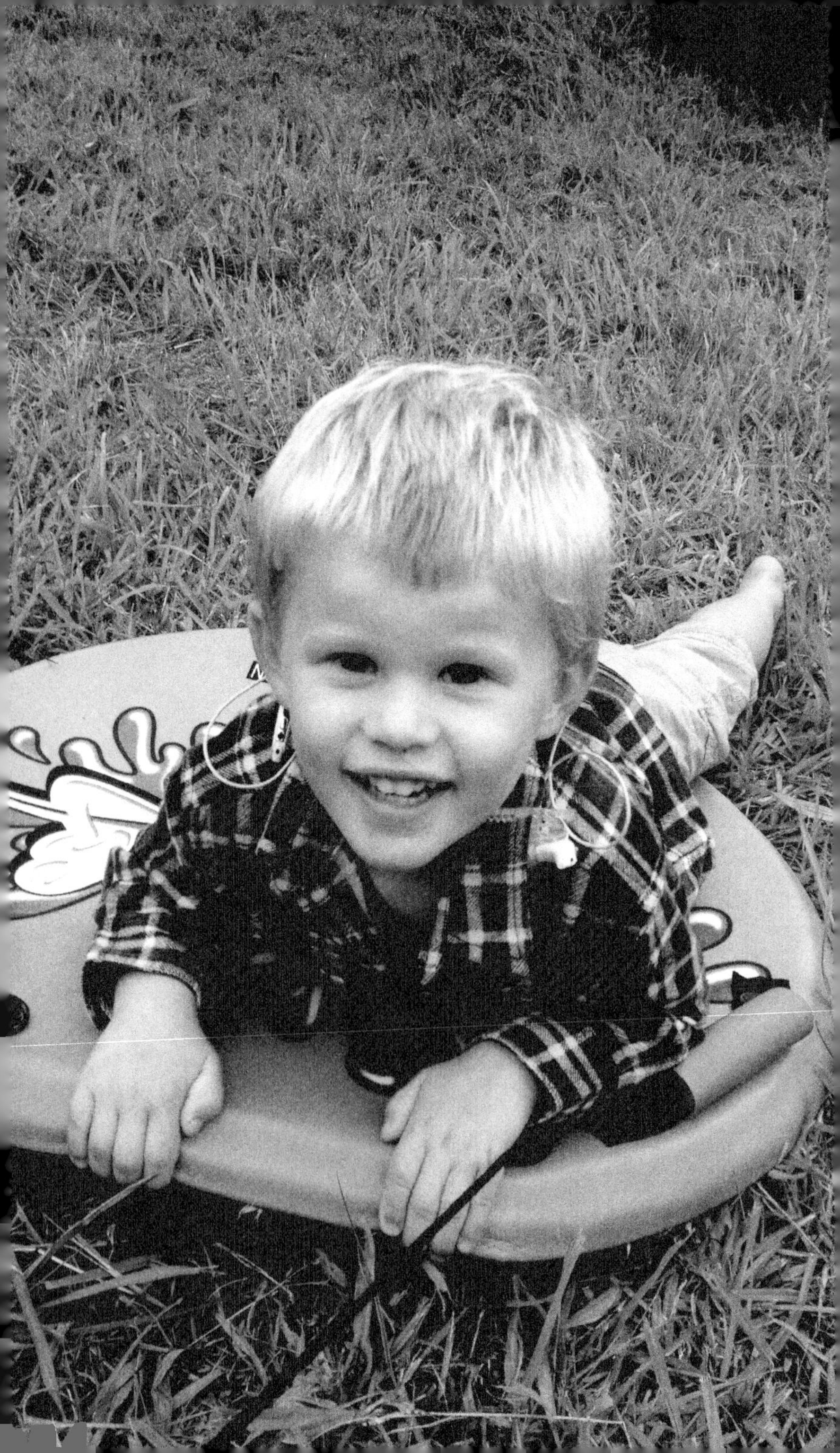

## *Sam's story*

# He's just Sam

*Language, sounds and language therapy are everywhere! It's not a one-hour session per day with specific toys and sounds - it's about building listening and speech therapy into everything you do. Every moment is an opportunity for you to teach and for your child to learn! Realising this was my real a-ha moment.*

*I was the mum completely tearing my hair out and feeling like a complete failure because my boy wouldn't do a daily home 'therapy' session with me from my special listening box, filled with the special toys I'd rushed out to buy because that's what I thought we 'needed' and what we used in Auditory Verbal therapy sessions at The Hearing House. The reality was he simply wasn't interested in sitting still or structured play; he was, and still is, an adventure kid!*

*While hanging out the washing one day, with Sam sitting in the washing basket handing me pegs, I realised this right here was a 'therapy' moment – "the peg is green"... "it goes up - up - up"... "thank you, Sam"... "one more for Mum". It was like a lightbulb moment. From that day on, I don't think we ever used the therapy box or prepared for a daily home therapy session ever again... I simply built therapy into our everyday life the Auditory Verbal way! And it worked!*

*Trust me when I say that when you hear that first or next word that you have worked so hard for your child to say, you appreciate it so, so, so much more!*

---

In 2008, little Sam (5.12 lbs) blessed our world, entering with a super quick labour and like Batman with one arm above his head. Little did we know this superpower attitude was going to be needed from us all for much bigger reasons than we could imagine at the time.

Our happy-go-lucky wee boy, nothing fazed him, he never cried, was always happy and busy and would sleep like you wouldn't believe, anywhere and through anything.

In the new year of 2010, life for a one-year-old was relatively straightforward and simple. I was a very young mum and we were just navigating life as first-time parents. Newborn hearing tests were not a thing and in our naivety about what Sam should and shouldn't be doing, we had no reason to even think to check. Even though I did have that boy who wouldn't engage at 'Wriggle and Rhyme' and wouldn't sit in one place, a hearing loss didn't occur to me. To be honest, he was a total nightmare at the session and, walking out of there, I decided that we were never going back again. Not long after that, I figured out why! Looking back, there are many of these 'oh that makes sense now' moments that family, friends and I can share – even Sam sleeping through a fire alarm!

And so the story begins...

One day we were asked by Sam's Grandma, "Do you think Sam is hearing?"

My instant reaction was to think, *don't be so stupid, of course he can hear,* but it planted the seed. After some basic

DIY testing such as calling Sam's name from behind him, making loud bangs, clapping behind his head (I'm not sure if I banged pots together too but it's very possible!), I was desperate for him to hear these sounds, but it was pretty obvious he wasn't - he was just a nosey, busy, searchy kid, fooling us and making his way in the world in complete silence.

This prompted a visit to the doctor, followed by a private ENT appointment to avoid long waiting lists. From there we were referred to Auckland Hospital for auditory brainstem response testing, where they measured the way Sam's brain reacted to sounds – this was the first of four general anaesthetic procedures Sam would undergo over the next twelve months.

Being told for the first time that we have a profoundly deaf child left us feeling like our world had been turned upside down. Unfortunately, the news wasn't delivered to us in the most caring way either. It was very matter of fact with no 'what happens next' (well, maybe there was but in the moment there was no info that I heard anyway), and we were just in complete shock. *What did this mean for our family, for our boy now ? A life of sign language? How would we navigate that?*

I remember Sam's dad and I coming home and standing in the kitchen of our cosy wee first home and just feeling numb. There were no words, and no actions in that moment that we could embrace to make it better.

That was until we met the crew at The Hearing House – this became the place of HOPE, of safety, the place where the answers and reassurance came from. The place where we were surrounded by others who 'got it', families going through the same emotional rollercoaster ride, professionals who could state the facts but also share other families' journeys. Our Auditory Verbal therapist, Estelle, was also a mum who understood exactly how we were feeling - she had a deaf son herself and so knew what we were dealing with - she taught me a lot!

It was here we also learnt that sign language wasn't necessary at this point. We were reminded that the biggest thing we could teach Sam now was to listen. An example I remember is this: 'If you're in France and only speak a few French words and you ask for directions, you'll listen hard. However, if someone points left or right and speaks at the same time, you will simply take the easy option and watch the hand signals'. Even now that Sam has been offered to learn sign language, he doesn't want to; he can hear, he just isn't interested.

So we learnt what a cochlear implant was; we'd never even heard of this technology before, let alone knew of anyone with one. I recall a really special moment when I met another child who was at The Hearing House at the same time as us. He was about seven – he could hear me! And speak! It was amazing! This made it real! This made the hope for Sam real!

From here, I don't think Sam's dad and I even discussed what was to happen next for Sam; together we just knew we wanted to give him the chance to function in a hearing world, to have the chance to experience the gift of a life of sound.

May 2010, Sam was implanted with his first cochlear implant – a device that converts sound waves to electrical impulses, then sends them to the brain. Who even comes up with this idea?! And then makes it a reality? Thank you Dr Graeme Clarke for your vision, talent and commitment to your idea; we are incredibly grateful. It changes lives, it changed our boy's life and ours too.

Now for the switch-on of 'Sam's Ears', as we still call them to this day. Back then, switch-on was three weeks post-surgery. We were told by the audiology team it would go one of three ways – happiness, tears or nothing. We wanted one of the first two and, boy, did we get it.

Switch-on was nothing like the YouTube videos, which you see of a baby smiling after hearing their mum's voice for the first time. For us, it was a mix of overwhelming and opposing emotions. Sam was traumatized – he was scared, we could see it in his eyes; this was the first time he was exposed to sound – from silence for over one and a half years to suddenly hearing something. He hated it, he screamed and cried and wasn't having a bar of this thing on his head or these sounds in his brain. We hated seeing him like this, but the conflicting thing was, we were also so happy to see it had worked – there again was HOPE. Some tweaks later and some serious persuasion, we got him out into the playground where he could move and play: he tolerated it for a wee while. I never actually watched Sam's first video and believe I even threw it away. It had been so distressing.

Then, the real fun began – Sam didn't want to wear his processor! It was so big on his little head and he didn't realise the sound value yet. We had these funny little hats (bonnets) we would put on him to try and get him to keep it on. Distraction, perseverance and some bribery at times too was key to winning the battle. Once he started to realise the benefits of wearing it, it was easy(ish) to get him to keep it on.

The next dark cloud over our heads was deciding if we could fund the 50K for surgery costs and a second implant for Sam (back then bilateral implants weren't funded), knowing that in this case two is better than one (after all, we were created with two ears for a reason).

One day, I called out to Sam from my bedroom window;

I could tell he could hear my voice as he stopped what he was doing but he couldn't find where the sound was coming from. He searched around but, with only one 'ear', couldn't pinpoint my location.

So, with family and friends we embarked on a fundraising journey to get the 50K we needed. Back then (I feel like I'm writing about the dinosaur ages but it was only twelve years ago), social media wasn't a big thing, neither were GoFundMe pages. We hosted lots of different events to fundraise, auctioned off donated goods and received many financial donations. It also unexpectedly increased awareness of cochlear implants in our community as we were interviewed for local papers a few times as well. It was a big task; it took us about eight months. People and businesses were so generous with their time, money and support. Saying thanks was the hardest thing. A 'thank you' never really felt like it was enough acknowledgement to show how much we appreciated everyone's support and the difference they were making to Sam's future.

I can recall the first time I had to speak publicly about Sam's journey, I couldn't do it - it was too raw, too painful. I started my speech and couldn't finish it, and the rest of the event was a blur for me. Come the next event, I shook like crazy with nerves but finished reading my speech word for word. A few events later, I could rattle off our story without paper and without a fear of public speaking. A life journey for me too!

I know that nowadays it's no longer necessary for families in New Zealand to have to do all this to raise money, and I'm so glad it's not! I cried the day that funding for bilateral implants was announced. Parents can now just be parents and focus on the development of their baby without this pressure.

The reality was that these were just the first couple of big steps into a much larger picture. Man, it takes a village, on many different levels with many different things to offer, to help a deaf child learn to listen and speak. Some of that village changes as the journey goes on but the need for it never goes away. We have been so fortunate to have been, and still be, surrounded by so many people who care and support both Sam and us: family, friends, professionals, teachers, to name just a few.

Sam's dad and I worked a lot, so we knew it was important to have Sam in an environment of learning and social skills development. Four days per week, he was in a great daycare with staff who really cared about him. More challenges came to light with learning, language delays and behaviour (yes, our frustrated boy was the classroom biter). Then we realised it was all too much for him, so we decided to break up the days. He attended home-based learning two days per week with a devoted and passionate lady. She gave the time and commitment to teach him in a quiet environment. He would then go to daycare for the other two days as we knew that social skills development was super important too, as well as learning to cope in noisy environments.

Moving into primary school, Sam attended a very small school - I think the maximum number of students was three hundred kids, including both primary and intermediate. This saw Sam continue to come forward in leaps and bounds – he didn't get lost, he had amazing teachers who cared and was supported in his learning with teacher aides.

Sam has always been about a year and a half behind his peers in learning and social skills. Over the past two years, the gap has started to narrow. Now he's in his early teens and more interested in learning about things.

Last year Sam was 'thrown into the frying pan' when

together we decided to send him to a boarding school. We're a year in now and we all know, including Sam, that this was the best move for him. He's making good friends, making smart life choices, has become so much more independent and is again supported by a brilliant learning support group and a team that are committed to 'growing great men'.

Throughout this, as much as the mum in me wanted to, we never wrapped Sam in cotton wool. He wanted to play rugby; I wanted him to play a safer sport, but my dad reminded me that he was a pretty stubborn boy and that if he wanted to play rugby, I wouldn't get him to play soccer! So he now plays rugby, cricket and social hockey. He manages just fine with protective headgear and one 'ear' on. He has climbed trees, played in the water, ridden his bikes and scooter, laughed, joked, played and just lived the most normal life we could give him.

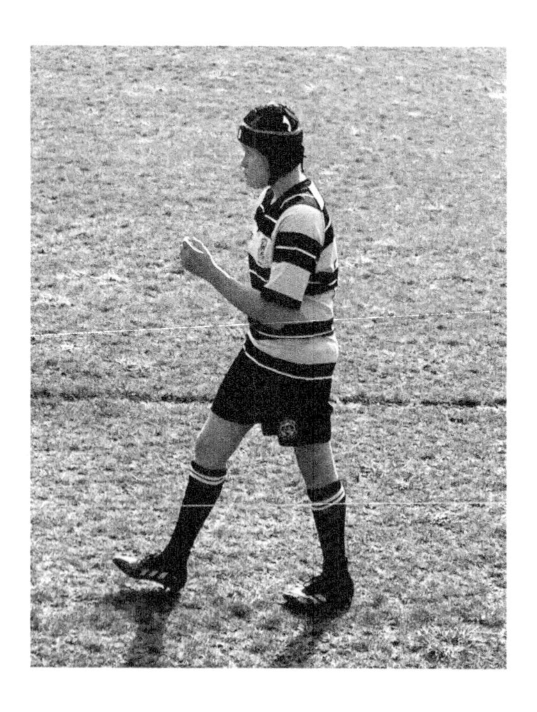

Parenting a child with cochlear implants comes with many interesting moments, some funny, some happy and some tough ones too. To share just a few:

- Once Sam was in the playground when one curious kid asked what they were. We just said they are Sam's special ears. The kid ran off to his mum saying, "I want some of those!".

- One day we were having a disagreement about something, Sam flicked his 'ears' off so he couldn't hear me – he only ever did that once as I took them off him and refused to communicate with him for a while (tough love, I know, but it worked!).

- As Sam got older and could self-manage his devices, I used to find myself every morning saying, "Sam where are your ears?!" or "Why do you only have one on?". Now he just gets 'the mum look' and knows.

For the most part, we have been very fortunate that most of his peers are totally understanding and accepting of Sam and his 'ears'. Ever-changing technology helps too – it's not odd for things to be in people's ears these days. Sam always just 'got on with it' so he's rarely experienced any bullying. We always made sure we gave Sam the confidence in himself and tools to deal with these situations.

I can't say it's all been a peachy journey; it's been hard. There have been moments of complete frustration, misunderstanding, shock. At times, he's been spoilt or we've tried to overcompensate for his differences (trust me, this doesn't work). There have been battles and big life changes, but with hard work, lots of talking, at times consequences and of course love, we continue to make it through together and I'm so incredibly proud of the young man Sam is becoming.

I asked Sam while I was writing this if he could tell me what it's like for him having cochlear implants, to which he replied, "I don't know" - a typical Sam answer but it's also in a way reassuring that this is just his normal life.

So, in closing, I'll say we don't know why Sam was born deaf and that's okay. But I think it's fair to say now that our world was never 'upside down' - it was simply on a wonky rotation and probably always will be, but this is our world, our journey and this is our boy - we don't ever look at Sam as a deaf child anymore. He's not, he's Sam, our happy-go-lucky, sports-mad, mainstreamed, caring and handsome young superman!

---

*My advice to anyone reading this is take everything you can get, talk to as many people as you can, educate, learn, fight the battles when you need to. To get the best for your child, listen to your gut and never forget that every moment is a learning moment.*

## *Nathan's story*

# A new life in a different world

The walls closed in. Time slowed. My pulse raced, yet my feet were leaden. Every step felt in slow motion, as if my feet were dragging in tar. The corridor called to me and yet seemed to be endlessly moving away like an ever-opening telescope. Cogent thought didn't come to me easily as I grappled with the tiny image unfolding at the corridor's end. It took all my effort to move towards something I didn't want to face. His hospital bed was to the left of this tiny image, its corners neatly folded and a heavy woollen blanket laying over the end of it, unused. No longer affording warmth. As I moved slowly forward, the sterile, shiny white tiles of the corridor seemed to envelop me. A cold emptiness swept over me, gnawing at me like hunger, my stomach gripped with fear. I had never known fear like it - something I didn't want to face but knew I had to. *Where was my boy?*

Slumped forward in the hospital armchair like a ragdoll, my husband Graham was sobbing uncontrollably. I knew in that moment that I would never be able to unsee this image. As I got nearer the room, I was numb with fear that Nathan was dead. There was a moment of silence as an ice fist seemed to grip my throat and my cracked voice screamed,

"Where is he? ...Where's my baby?"

In that moment, no thought of 'our' baby; he was mine, born of my body, my joy, my responsibility. My husband's steel blue eyes looked up at me, every conflicting emotion reflected there. In the silence, I heard my own heartbeat insistent in my ears.

"It was awful, I...," he hesitantly began.

My unfeeling voice cut through his need, "Where *IS* he?"

"In Intensive Care."

Now there was a rift between us. A rift I had unknowingly created. An inability to see his pain or acknowledge his need in that moment. It wasn't that I didn't care, there was just no room in my consciousness to consider him. We were both gripped by fear and desperation but unable to unite within it. All I thought was that I needed to be with my son. Abandoning my husband with no thought for his pain, I ran from the ward down the corridor to ICU with a surge of potential hope in my heart... he was still alive.

My mind was in turmoil trying to understand just what had happened and how he could have left our baby alone in ICU. How could he feel like that and sit in the empty ward, when these may be the last precious moments that we had with our son? I judged him as weak and had no reserves to support him. I needed to immerse myself in the reality of the moment to cope. He needed to distance himself from it, to avoid its reality. Action was my saviour, denial was his. We all cope with trauma in our own ways and, with time to reflect, we can appreciate another's pain. But, in that moment, I could not. Later, I found out that Graham had been with him when he had stopped breathing and had tried to resuscitate him, keeping him alive long enough for the hospital staff to run down the corridor to his bedside. Now, he couldn't face any more.

In ICU, the tiny motionless body of my son lay in the

hospital cot with wires on his chest and forehead, their monitors bleeping, their lights reassuring me that there was still hope. I reached out to hold his tiny fingers and the warmth of his hand began to abate my fear. My eyes flickered between his face and the machine traces that kept his life in the balance. I'm not sure how long I had sat there before a muted voice whispered at the periphery of my world, breaking into our bubble. The doctor needed information. I can't recall the questions he asked or the answers I gave but he reassured me that Nathan was stable for now. Staff came and went, measuring his temperature, checking his pulse, and altering his fluids. I still didn't know what had happened or why he was here.

As the staff worked, my mind drifted back to just twelve hours earlier when I had woken to Nathan's strange unrecognizable screams in the middle of the night. I had lifted him from his cot to nurse him and realised that he had a raging temperature. I tried Calpol but couldn't settle him, then he was sick and began to cough up blood. We rang for an ambulance. During the frightening drive over Sha Tin Mountain, my mind was awhirl with memories from my childhood. It is strange how childhood memories flood your consciousness when a crisis happens. My own mother had been a fever nurse and I remembered her worrying about symptoms like very high temperatures, unusual screaming and sickness as signs of meningitis. Is that what this was? No one was telling me anything. I felt my anxiety rising again. I didn't want to leave Nathan's side to find the doctor to ask about my fears. My husband joined me, and I asked him to go and find someone who could answer our questions.

A tall, heavily-built consultant came to the bedside and I shared my fears. He dismissed them, saying I had let Nathan get seriously dehydrated and that was the issue. I knew this wasn't true. We had lived here in Hong Kong for a year, and I had always taken great care to ensure Gemma and Nathan were well hydrated throughout the day. I knew this wasn't right, but how do you argue with a consultant when you don't know what is happening yourself? I wondered how many other parents had had their fears dismissed like this. Nathan was still unconscious and not responding to my voice at all, and it seemed that the consultant was dismissing me as a mother who had not taken care of her child. Several hours passed and still Nathan showed no signs of response. It was late at night now and clearly the consultant had finished for the day. A young registrar put his head around the door of ICU, and I shouted at him, "Please listen to me! My son is not dehydrated or if he is, it's not because of lack of water. Something is desperately wrong... Something inside me knows he is dying."

He gave me time to explain my fears, listened and said he would do further tests. He asked Graham to go with him to fill out permission slips. I later found out he wanted to talk to him about whether I was always so hyper-anxious and unreasonable about the children's health. Graham told him he had never seen me like this and the doctor responded that they might have missed something. A doctor who respected a parent's fears at last! To this day, I feel that this young doctor was the one who saved Nathan's life.

Just fifteen minutes later, I was tightly gripping the rail of Nathan's cot as it was pushed towards the huge swing doors of the hospital theatre. I was semi-conscious of Graham walking with me, a gulf of fear and tension in the air. Nathan needed a lumber puncture, the registrar feared meningitis. As we both struggled with the emotions of knowing our one-year-old needed a needle in his spine, we were wrenched back to the moment by Nathan's cries. A nurse was struggling to restrain him in a foetal position to give the doctor access to his spinal column. His spine needed to be absolutely still for the needle insertion, but he was resisting. The more tightly she held him, the more he screamed. I couldn't bear to hear him, and my maternal instinct was to push the nurse aside and cradle him, but I wasn't sure what to do for the best. Then, sensing my anxiety, the young doctor asked if I would like to try. I curled my son's body under my own like a warm cocoon leaving only his back exposed. I closed my eyes and held my breath, mustering as much courage and strength as I could as the needle plunged between his vertebrae. He tried to arch away from me, screaming violently, but the procedure was done. I opened my eyes, looking but not wanting to see as the cloudy white fluid was slowly drawn from his spine. I saw a knowing glance between the doctor and the nurse, and I knew.

The fluid needed to be cultured but they began antibiotic treatment immediately in preparation for a positive diagnosis of bacterial meningitis. This was just the beginning of a journey for our family of fighting to be heard and supporting our boy through profound deafness, which was the undiagnosed legacy of the meningitis.

Nathan was now in a coma being monitored hourly and wired to a plethora of machines, which flashed and bleeped, reinforcing in my mind that he still might not make it. They struggled to get a line in to enable a steady flow of drugs and finally had to insert into a vein in his forehead. I am not sure why, but this was such a shock for me, seeing my little man with a tube secured to the front of his head. It somehow made it even more real and his hold on life so tenuous. They regularly tested for responses under the arch of his foot and on his cheek, but nothing. He was breathing on his own and that was the single fact I held onto. Another lumber puncture was done to see if the antibiotics were taking effect, but the fluid was still cloudy. The consultant who had previously ignored my concerns would not speak with me at all and the conversations were all held with the nurses almost acting as translators. Daily I asked them if Nathan would wake up, knowing they couldn't answer me; it was just a waiting game.

Then about two weeks later, Nathan began to stick his tongue between his lips in a comforting habit I recognised immediately. I sat by his bed and held his hand, talking to him and praying that he would open his eyes. The young registrar reassured me that, if I felt this was a habit he had before meningitis, it could be a good sign that he would wake up soon, but he wasn't certain. A day or two later, Nathan woke. We still didn't know if there was brain damage or any permanent disability, but he was going to live.

We had been in intensive care for over three weeks and after his illness, he could no longer walk or talk and was so weak I had to carry him like a baby in my arms. His eyes were still bright and focused and so I felt strongly that he hadn't suffered brain damage - but why wasn't he speaking or listening to me? He used few of the words he had known before his illness and he still cried violently when I was out of sight.

At least we were able to take him home. After a few hours at home, I began to wonder if he was hearing me. Sometimes I thought he was because he responded with a smile or a gesture, but he didn't turn when I called him. It was all so confusing! Was he just weak and traumatised by his illness or was it something more? That night when he was asleep, I took a metal spoon and saucepan and banged it violently near him... NO response! He couldn't hear!

So, back to the hospital next day. I knew that the senior consultant wouldn't listen to me so instead of going to reception, I walked the wards trying to find the young doctor who had trusted me. Over the years to come, that would be my strategy: to waste no time with professionals who didn't listen. Nathan's time was too precious to waste. Little did I know at this time that most of the professionals who would come into our lives would tell me what Nathan couldn't do, rather than what was possible.

Graham found it hard to accept that the consultants might be wrong but was always supportive and 'had my back' when I questioned a doctor. Perhaps his structured military view of the world made him implicitly trust authority, but my own mother who was a nurse had always told me to question doctors if you didn't agree. She had worked with health professionals all her life and always said there are good and bad listeners, as in all walks of life, and this sustained me when I had to advocate for my son. I am sure I was often labelled as a 'difficult mother', but I didn't care - I just wanted the best possible outcome for my son. This registrar at least had listened!

So, the testing began. Unfortunately, I had to meet again with the senior consultant who had been so curt and unfeeling with me before. He sat Nathan in a small baby chair and shook a tin of marbles behind him. Nathan turned.

The consultant looked at me and said, "Your son can hear; he is just traumatised by his illness."

He wouldn't refer him for further testing. At this time, we didn't know that hearing loss could be caused by meningitis.

At home, I saw no responses and still believed Nathan couldn't hear. There was no internet to search for information so I researched at the library and found out that meningitis could damage children's hearing. I was convinced that Nathan's hearing had been wiped out completely. I rang a close friend in London who I knew had a sister on the Bart's

Hospital staff and asked where the best place was to take our son for a full hearing assessment. She recommended the Royal National Hospital in London. We began to plan a visit to the UK and waited to hear about an appointment.

A couple of weeks later, we were walking down the street and I was carrying Nathan on my left hip with my face close to his right ear. Graham was walking ahead with our daughter, Gemma. I shouted loudly for them to wait for us and, as I did so, Nathan turned to face me. Had he heard my voice? Or just felt the vibrations of my shout? I wasn't sure, so I put my mouth to his ear and loudly said, "Give Mummy a kiss." He looked at me blankly, no response. Perhaps I had just imagined it, and my heart sank. As Graham approached, I told him what had happened. Then he laughed and said, "Ask him to smack me, he might do that!" Again, I shouted into Nathan's ear, "Give Daddy a smack." This time he reached out and smacked his father... I couldn't believe that he had responded! There was some hope that he could hear! Maybe he had a little hearing after all... light at the end of my tunnel.

Shortly after that, I flew back to London to see Specialist Consultant, Dierdre Lucas, at the Royal National Hospital and get a second opinion. The army would not release Graham to come with me, so I had to fly alone with both children. Poor Gemma was only three years old and had her world turned upside down - her parents almost permanently at the hospital, all the family talking constantly of Nathan and now flying fourteen hours to London with us. She was to be her brother's biggest advocate and support in the years to come.

Dr Lucas's team confirmed that Nathan had no useable hearing in his left ear and only a low frequency corner audiogram at profound levels in his right. He was duly fitted with one body-worn hearing aid. The advice was that he would not ever be able to hear speech or learn to speak. Despite what I had experienced, they felt that his responses were just vibrotactile (physical sensation response) and he was using the context of what he had known before to make sense of requests. It felt like we were back at the beginning again. Perhaps they were right and he couldn't hear speech at all, just rhythm of sound.

And so, our journey began. I didn't know what the options were for our son, but I knew I wanted him to speak, if at all possible. I also knew that almost everyone told us that wasn't a possibility, so I began a course in British Sign Language. If this needed to be the path we were to follow, I would be ready, but I didn't sign with Nathan. I really, really hoped that he could be part of our hearing, speaking family. I knew that my parents and extended family would not be able to learn to sign and it would be a challenge for all of us to be able to interpret Nathan's needs and wants for him in many situations. The mountain in front of us seemed insurmountable and I cried myself to sleep many nights.

When I was trying to find out more information about routes of communication we could look at, I remembered from university that a man called Daniel Ling had taught profoundly deaf children to speak using lip-reading and making use of any minimal residual hearing they might have. So, I enrolled in a university course to learn more. I knew nothing about cochlear implants as they were in their infancy in UK in the eighties and Nathan was not eligible because of his age and lack of spoken language. Those were the criteria at the time. Our army life also made it difficult to advocate for services as we moved house so frequently.

Then our luck changed when we moved to Catterick in northern England. We were given a teacher of the deaf who listened to what I hoped and dreamed of for our son. She counselled me that, in her professional opinion, Nathan would never speak but, that said, she would support me in whatever choice I made. Over the next year, we worked together to try and make a link between the words Nathan had in his head from hearing until he was eighteen months old and the patterns on my lips. As he slowly recovered physically from his illness and learned to walk again, his concentration span began to improve. It was very slow and very challenging but gradually he began to respond when we spoke to him. He also began to use again a few of the words he had before losing his hearing and slowly communication was re-established. Once he understood what was needed, he sought out lip patterns from everyone and began to make sense of his world. His speech would be difficult to understand for anyone outside the family for several more years, but we persevered and, as hearing aid

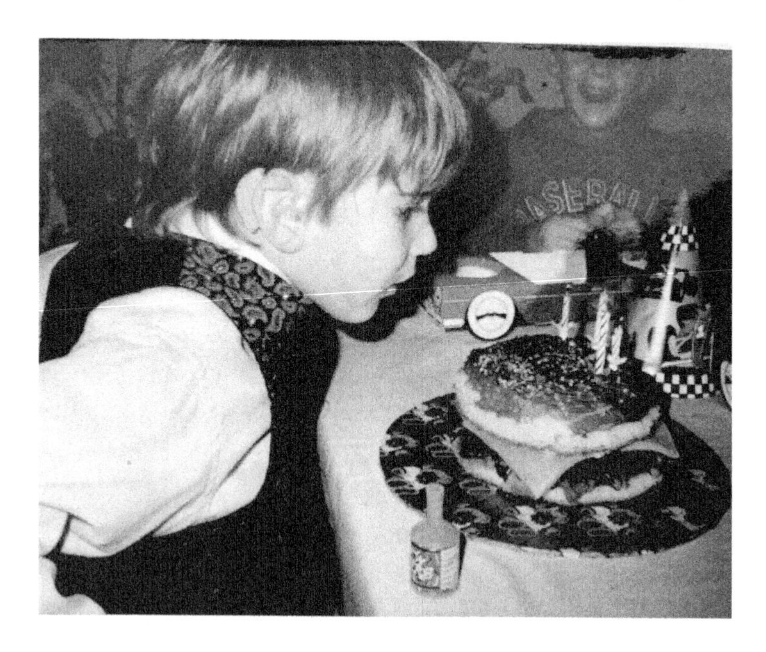

technology improved, he began to make more responses to sound supported by lip-reading.

Reading books was his lifesaver and was to be his solace throughout his schooling when times were challenging both academically and socially. By the time he went to school, he could point to the words in books correctly. Although his pronunciation was often awry, I knew he was reading in his head. His sister, Gemma, was a wonderful support for him in school; being only one year above, she was regularly sent for to interpret what Nathan was trying to say in the first couple of years of his schooling. She was patient and caring with him and often read to him at home and taught him new words, even though she was only six years old. Even his little brother Adam knew to face him when speaking and often helped him by repeating things people said. Gradually, Nathan's language and speech skills developed. Again, the school and professionals told me it was the wrong thing to do to correct his speech or his attempts at new words as it would undermine his confidence and slow his progress. This didn't sit well with me, and I felt he needed to hear and lipread the correct models to be able to improve his speech. I introduced a Sooty hand puppet so that when errors occurred, I could tell Sooty to try again and Nathan loved to take his puppet everywhere, often telling him off by wagging his finger at him and saying "again". I really feel that helped him to speak more clearly.

It was difficult getting support for Nathan throughout his schooling as, being an army family, we moved houses constantly and each time we needed to explain to schools that, despite him being profoundly deaf, we wanted our son to speak not sign, and that he would need support. Again, I was often seen as 'difficult', pushing for support when they felt sign would have given him a language more quickly, but we persevered and slowly Nathan's speech became more comprehensible.

When Nathan was seven, we moved to an army base in Wiltshire where we found an amazing primary school, Christ The King. The staff there were so supportive and raised expectations for Nathan to communicate and speak more clearly. He had fulltime support from a wonderful teaching assistant, Trisha Martin, who worked with him daily to improve his speech and help access information in the classroom. Again, his love of books sustained him in his learning through primary school. It was only later that I realised going to the library was also a way he avoided difficult social interaction in the playground. Trisha became a huge part of our lives, always willing to chat and, most importantly, she listened to what we wanted for our son.

There were many challenges and hurdles to overcome throughout Nathan's schooling, mostly with schools lowering expectations because of his deafness or suggesting that he was doing so well 'for a deaf child'. He went on to be very successful academically, but the social side of his life was always a challenge. It was so difficult to be part of noisy boisterous teenage banter when he needed to lip-read everyone's contribution.

At age eighteen, Nathan was accepted at university but after a year he found the environment too challenging with no hearing. We were lucky enough to find a surgeon who was prepared to risk cochlear implant surgery on one of his ears despite all medical indications to the contrary. So, after a two-year funding wait, Nathan was successfully implanted at twenty and began Auditory Verbal Therapy to hear for the first time in nineteen years.

It is a hard thing to watch your child struggle, realising you don't have all the answers but neither do the professionals.

*'Trust your instincts and listen to those who listen to you'* became my self-mantra.

I will just close by saying it was a tough journey for Nathan, but his determination and resilience have seen him through many challenges, failures, and prejudices. I am so proud of the man he has become and that he is now giving back to the deaf and hard of hearing community as an audiologist.

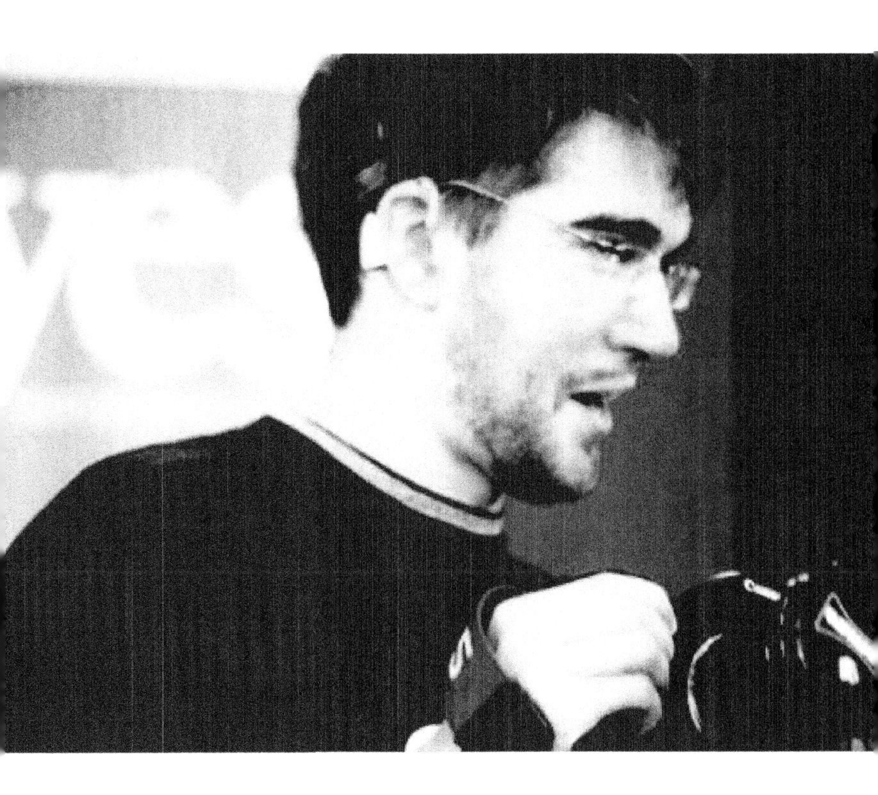

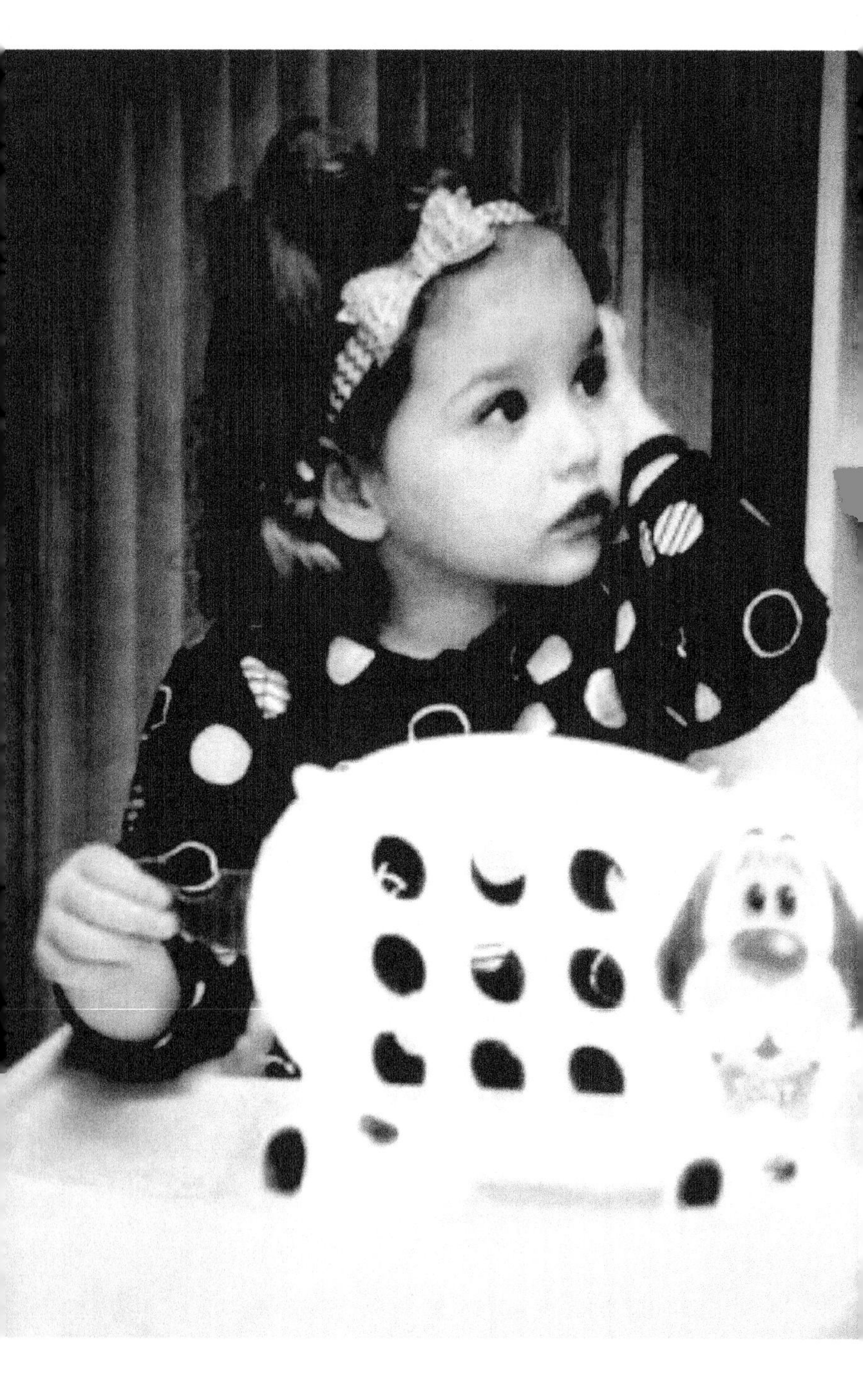

*Poppy's story*

# Through Poppy's eyes

We spent hours and hours holding our sweet girl with the longest eyelashes in one of the sound-proofed rooms at Waikato Hospital. We took turns holding her carefully not to disturb her or the many wires attached to her head, unable to speak to each other but deeply worried by what the outcome could be.

Being told the news that she had hearing loss in both ears was a shock to us, but we naively held onto the fact that she had some hearing and that hearing aids would do the trick. We reassured ourselves that it was *just* a hearing loss, and we could manage the hearing aids. We knew nothing of the impact that this hearing loss diagnosis was to have on our lives, or the complications of the more complex further diagnoses that awaited us.

We persevered with hearing aids for the next twelve months and Poppy failed every test, every one. Each time we hoped for answers, and I repeatedly asked if Poppy's hearing loss could be progressive. I was told it was unlikely. We were seeing no responses at home and our worry and frustration were building. It became so obvious to me that these hearing aids were useless and finally after many, many heartbreaking visits to audiology, Poppy was scheduled for further testing under general anaesthetic.

After a long wait, we were called into one of those little

hospital rooms. The look on the audiologist's face said it all, and then the words, "Poppy has a profound hearing loss in both ears."

It was in that moment that I cried uncontrollably. The world of my precious little girl had been shattered. The audiologist hurried out of the room, bringing in someone more senior to console me... who blurted out that there are plenty of deaf children who lead great lives. In that moment, amongst all the noise, that was of little comfort to me.

This was the moment that began our long and challenging journey to teach our baby Poppy to listen and speak.

After Poppy's diagnosis a dark cloud of worry followed me constantly... questions raged in my mind:

*How will we communicate with her?*

*Will she have friends?*

*How will she get on at school?*

*How will she play sport?*

Things moved very quickly from here and, through the fog, I am grateful that I documented it all. It proved to be very therapeutic, and I am thankful that I had the foresight.

We were contacted only a few days later by The Hearing House. We were to meet to discuss the assessment process and what would be involved should Poppy be able to receive cochlear implants.

Mark and I felt overwhelmed, we were still in shock. We knew nothing about implants or deafness. I was in a constant state of worry. At times I look back at those early days, feeling hard done by, robbed of a lot of the joy of having my beautiful child. In hindsight, it was good that we had little time to dwell on it, or fear and worry may have paralyzed us. We knew without much discussion that we wanted Poppy to have the best chance of being able to listen and speak. If we could make that decision for her and it was possible, we would do whatever it took to make it happen.

We made the trip to Auckland from Hamilton. We found it confronting, there was no sugar coating. This was going to take a lot of dedication and hard work. We had to show we were committed to the process of travelling to Auckland each week and putting in the necessary work. Little did we know that this process would prove to be much harder and longer than most. We also had to consider our older daughter, Lily, who was almost four at the time, but we knew that we would find a way to make it work.

After all the tests, assessments, MRI scans, etc. had been done, it was crunch time and we handed Poppy over to the nurse (she was just fourteen months old). She smiled back at us in her little scrubs and bounced along, holding onto the nurse's whites, down the corridor and into theatre, completely oblivious to the life-changing surgery she was about to undergo.

We had met with Estelle before Poppy's surgery and had done a session or two of Auditory Verbal Therapy to get into the groove of what our weekly sessions would be like. Estelle was Poppy's Auditory Verbal therapist and proved to be an integral part of Poppy's journey.

At the time, I was a stay-at-home mum. Mark and I had both made the commitment that we would attend every session together. So, every Friday we drove to Auckland and attended the one-hour session. We learnt about the Ling sounds and putting listening first. Everything was foreign to us, we had to get out of our comfort zone, but we loved those sessions. Even a turn of the head as Poppy responded to sound was exciting progress and we tried to soak up any information we could and put in the hard yards at home.

The burden of responsibility weighed heavily on me as I was the one at home with Poppy during the day. I put enormous pressure on myself to ensure her speech and language developed. I came across a meme saying, 'A worried mother does better research than the FBI'. This was me to a tee; I would spend hours and hours on the internet trying to find other examples of children just like Poppy.

Just before Poppy's surgery and after the MRI, it was discovered that the most probable cause of Poppy's deafness was Cytomegalovirus or CMV for short. This was a huge worry for us and, as time went on and Poppy's progress continued to be a lot slower than the average, we became concerned that perhaps our end goal of spoken language was not going to be possible. The CMV had really complicated the picture.

As Poppy approached her third birthday, it was a particularly challenging time for us. We were battling with parent guilt, trying to make sure our eldest daughter was also well cared for and had allocated undivided attention while committing to Poppy's ongoing needs.

Poppy could understand most of what we were saying but only had a handful of words. Progress was so painfully slow.

Sport became a blessing in disguise for our little family. Mark and I both enjoyed team sports and wanted our girls to experience the fun and camaraderie that sport provides. Our eldest daughter, Lily, played Rippa Rugby from three years of age and as soon as Poppy turned three, she joined a team. This became a real social vehicle for Poppy. It didn't matter that she couldn't communicate with her peers; she could certainly pick up a ball and run with it, and she just loved it! Her big sister led the way and became a key role model for giving everything and anything a go.

Between ages three and four was really the hardest time. So much so that there were times I doubted my own ability and if I was made of the right stuff to see this through. It was a really hard phase of the journey. Many, many tears were shed.

We sought help from Diane Levy, a parenting coach. We attended a session at The Hearing House and then a private session at her house. I laugh when I think about it now, but Mark and I were really at our wits' end and went to great lengths to educate ourselves on how to parent this frustrated little human who just wanted to be heard but quite simply didn't have the language ability yet.

Poppy wasn't sleeping well at night, waking three or four times every night and becoming increasingly frustrated that she couldn't communicate her needs or wants. Poppy was attending several half days at kindy, and it was becoming more and more apparent how far behind her peers she was. We applied for an education support worker and Heather, the owner of the kindergarten, took on this role which provided Poppy with extra one-on-one support. We also applied for a Roger microphone for her teacher to use, which proved to be an essential tool.

Poppy is a strong-willed kid, who is relentlessly determined and, whilst this is a fantastic quality which will no doubt help her in life, it proved incredibly challenging during the phase I call 'threenager'. We left our weekly AVT sessions often quite despondent. Poppy was frustrated and over it, despite all the hard work Mark and I were putting in at home.

In the beginning we met other parents whose children were having remarkable success. Highflyers, I like to call them. "When the words come, they will not stop. You will be amazed," they said. "Once you hit ten words, the next month you will have a hundred and then sentences."

That was so hard to hear when Poppy's progress was so slow. When you are early in your journey, you hang on every expressive word. We just could not work out why our laborious efforts were not paying off. That was just not how it went at all for Poppy. We were lucky if she had ten solid words, some of which only we could understand. The vibe at home began to change. The option of sign language was tossed around more frequently, and we felt like our goal for Poppy learning to listen and speak was becoming out of reach. The fog began to set in, and I spent a lot of time agonizing if we were doing the right thing by pursuing spoken language.

Despite this, we persevered. Renique, a new therapist, took on Poppy for the final year before school. She was fresh out of training and was aware that Poppy was a special case. She really embraced the challenge and often spoke to Estelle for new ideas and techniques. This change sparked a new enthusiasm for Poppy. Mark and I again began to see little steps of progress. Although the sessions became enjoyable again, we knew that school was looming, and we knew that Poppy was nowhere near where she needed to be. We suspected that CMV was responsible for her slow progress and thought that she may have some sort of disorder like dyspraxia preventing her from advancing further.

Estelle suggested that we contact her friend Liz, a renowned Auditory Verbal therapist who had a practice at the University of Auckland specializing in articulation disorders. Liz had extensive knowledge and if anyone could provide answers, she was our lady.

Meeting Liz was a turning point. Mark and I sat there

in absolute amazement as Poppy attempted every sound that was asked of her and, after some practice and several attempts, was able to get lip closure to form "b" and said "bath" perfectly!

We sat there smiling like we had just won the lottery; this was something we had been trying for the last two and half years. Liz's excitement was infectious, and what she was able to achieve in one hour confirmed to us that spoken language for Poppy was possible.

We got to work. We made weekly appointments in Auckland with Liz and fortnightly appointments with Renique. These sessions complimented each other. Heather at kindy was also involved and regularly updated with sounds and words we were working on, and was so supportive of what we were trying to achieve.

It was not long after this that we had Julie come on board. A registered teacher of the deaf, her job was to educate the teachers and make sure Poppy had the adequate equipment and set-up for optimal learning. She also did one-on-one sessions twice a week with Poppy, something that continues to this day.

We continued to work hard – well, everyone did. We had a village of people who also wanted to see this kid fly. Four months before school started, we took up the challenge of applying for Ongoing Resourcing Scheme (ORS) funding. We were told by the Ministry of Education that Poppy wouldn't get it and very few deaf children in New Zealand do. We didn't listen and we persevered with the application anyway. We provided all the necessary paperwork and examples of why she needed it. Our village of audiologists, speech therapists, surgeons and teachers also helped with the mammoth application.

Lo and behold, she got it! This was a huge relief and a

real triumph. We knew that Poppy would be given the best possible chance of reaching her potential, whatever that looked like, and having additional teacher aide hours for her schooling life would be a tremendous help.

The first day of school came around and it wasn't without its challenges. Being able to craft friendships was one of the hardest aspects; with limited speech, it was very difficult.

The teachers were incredibly supportive and set up a buddy system which really helped. We continued to drive the three-hour round trip to Auckland every week for another three years. Poppy's speech and language continued to improve, the social part of school became more enjoyable, and she participated fully in all aspects of school life, taking on each challenge as it arose.

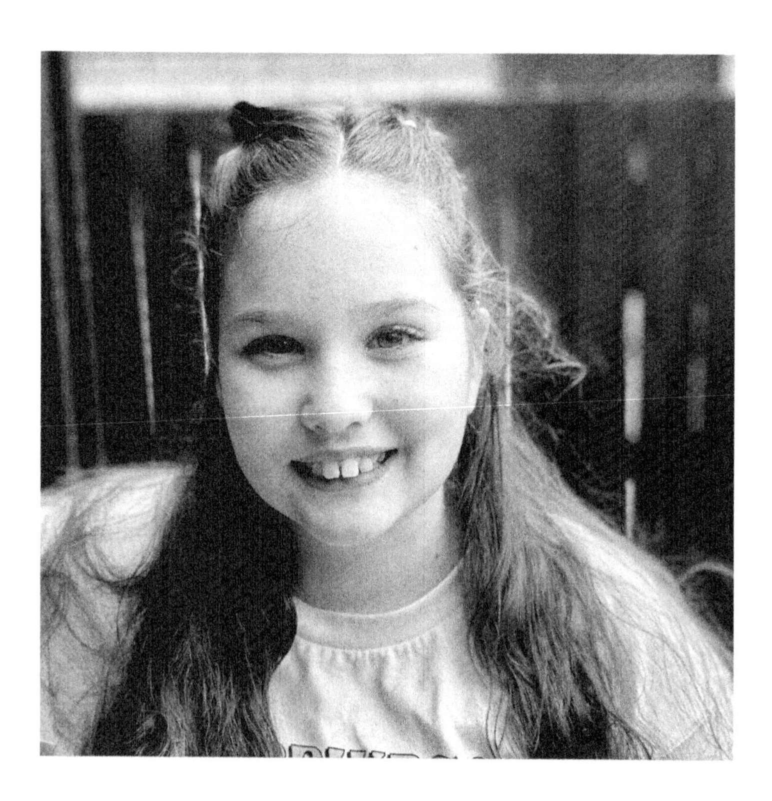

The last two years with COVID and home learning were particularly difficult, as it was for all children. There was no doubt that this disruption set Poppy back with her learning, but we are well and truly out the other side now.

Poppy is now nine years old and nearing the end of Year 4. This has been a great year for her and again she has come a long way at school, making incredible progress. This simply would not have been possible without the support of her amazing team whom we are lucky and so grateful to have.

Poppy enjoys basketball and soccer and although she finds schoolwork a challenge she enjoys learning and has many friends. We have no doubt that she will get there in her own sweet time as she has her entire life. She will continue to live life to the fullest and will never be defined by her deafness.

Last night we were all watching Home Alone, as you do at Christmas time. Poppy turned to me, looked me straight in the eyes, batting her long luscious lashes, and said, "Merry Christmas, Mumma."

It was so heartfelt and sincere and took me straight back to when she was a baby and when we both had so many fears for her future. *Would she ever be able to speak, would we ever have a moment like that?* The answer is clearly yes! I guess only parents with children with hearing loss can relate.

I am forever changed in that I will always recognise the magic moments in the everyday. I will never get tired of "Excuse me, Mum," or the Christmas carols sung completely off key, or the bellowing, "MUM... MUM, TOAST PLEASE!" so loud the neighbours can hear, but she can't because her 'ears' aren't on yet.

Or how she welcomes the neighborhood kids inside, kindly offering them cookies or any other treats she can find, and moves from room to room like a hurricane, but always making sure they are taken care of. Even though I'm out feverishly with the vacuum, a little miffed that I have to clean up, I know deep down that this is pretty cool, and things could have been so different.

Lily and Poppy's bond has evolved and at times they fight like cat and dog, but they have a friendship like no other. Lily is at that age when she asks questions, she wants to know why people are the way they are. My answer has and always will be that people with differences just want to be treated like everyone else. This year Lily's kindness at school has been recognized several times; she has a sensitive side that adults don't always see. I enjoy our little chats and I see her soaking in every word. I love that she does her thing quietly, not seeking attention or recognition, but genuinely just wanting to make people feel good.

Where am I going with this? I'm not really sure. I guess what I want to say is take time to recognize those magic moments if you're at the start of this journey, or even on a completely different one. There is magic in the everyday if you take the time to see it. Stick with it and it will come right.

Wishing you all good health, happiness and heaps of fun.

*Gunny's story*

# Unexpected new beginnings

I was eight and a half months pregnant and living in India. My husband, Raj, and I had planned everything to the last detail. We had made reservations at the local maternity hospital and even paid the advance - a requirement in India as otherwise hospitals run out of beds. I was counting days. I was soon going to have my baby. It was like the last lap. I couldn't wait.

I had taken an appointment with my gynaecologist for a routine ultrasound to ensure everything was going well. Raj was with me and we were waiting for our turn. Then suddenly, just out of the blue, Raj said something that left me a little shocked.

He asked, "Don't you think it would be better if we had our child in New Zealand?"

At first I thought he made that as a casual remark and, before I could react, we got called in.

The doctor performed the ultrasound. Everything was good and just when we were leaving the doctor's chamber, Raj asked the gynaecologist if she would give us a 'fit to fly certificate' if we wanted to travel to New Zealand to have our baby. I was quiet. I knew he was no longer joking. The doctor agreed saying that while she would not recommend flying at this late stage, if we were sure this is what we wanted to do, considering that my pregnancy had been 'uneventful' and everything was going well, she would give the certificate required to board an aircraft at this late stage of pregnancy.

All of a sudden, here we were talking about taking a flight in ten days' time to a country where we had no family, no relationships and where we had only spent two summers. I was nervous but at the same time, I started thinking about our new life in New Zealand. How exciting it would be! I had confidence in Raj's ability to work things out – the tickets, the rental apartment, appointments with the doctors once we landed, etc. I even requested my mother to fly with us for additional support. Even though she thought that the whole idea was a little crazy, she agreed to travel. We boarded a flight ten days later and flew half way across the world to have our baby and start a new life in New Zealand.

Surprisingly, it all seemed planned once we got to NZ. There was no trouble moving into our furnished rental apartment. I met with my local midwife clinic who got us appointments one after the other at Auckland Hospital so Baby's development could be checked. Ultrasounds and blood tests were done. My amniotic fluids were a little elevated and the doctors decided that the baby should be born at Auckland Hospital instead of Birth Care. I was given a date which was about two weeks out to check into the hospital for induced labour. When the day - July 25, 2012 - finally arrived, I checked into Auckland Hospital and Sunny was born close to midnight on the same day.

The next day around late morning, a nurse walked into my room pushing a trolley that carried a machine and said she wanted to perform a hearing test on Baby. I was exhausted and didn't have any energy to talk much or try and understand why the test was necessary. I let her get on with what she needed to do. She placed something that looked like headphones around Sunny's ears and a sensor on his forehead. In only a couple of minutes, she seemed done and left the room. Frankly I had no idea why this was necessary and really did not attach any importance to the test. I found out later that this was the standard newborn hearing screening test.

Having no one in our family with hearing loss, we had no reason to be concerned. It was only the next day when she came in again, wanting to repeat the test, that I sat up and took notice. This time I asked if the result was what she expected. To this, the nurse replied that she was not able to pick up any hearing and this most likely was on account of fluid in Baby's ears. Hence, we had nothing to worry about and she would come back again the next day to repeat the test. The third day when she was unable to detect any hearing, we got concerned. I think we were told at the time that it was still most likely fluid build-up in the ears preventing the test from showing any positive results. The nurse also informed us that she would schedule an advanced hearing examination called the ABR in about a month's time.

After three days when we finally got home, all Raj and I could think about was whether our baby could hear. This was our first child. We were trying to enjoy our baby. But Sunny having some sort of a disability was always at the back of our minds. It kept us in a constant state of worry and something that always kept the atmosphere tense at home in those early days. We tried not speaking about it much but we were both very anxious. We wanted the ABR to be expedited. Raj must have made a half a dozen phone calls to have it brought forward. Finally, after repeated follow ups, we were given an appointment four weeks later. Those were a very difficult four weeks. We were trying to stay as positive as we could, hoping and praying all along that it was in fact fluid in the ears and nothing serious.

On the day of the ABR, we reached Greenlane Hospital and were taken to a quiet insulated room by a senior audiologist. I was asked to sit in a chair and hold Sunny in my arms as the audiologist attached the many wires to his head and ears. The test started and seemed to go on forever. It was so hard to sit there and wait in uncertainty. Once the test concluded, the audiologist finally shared with us her findings. Sunny had "profound hearing loss in both ears".

Raj, holding back tears, asked what that really meant. The audiologist then went on to say that the profound nature of the hearing loss meant that Sunny was deaf. I couldn't stop myself, I burst out crying. Both Raj and I did. I felt as though my world had shattered right in front of my eyes. I had not experienced a bigger shock in my life. Until that day, we had never encountered a deaf person. I had a million questions running through my head. I wanted answers. *Would my baby ever be able to talk? Would I be able to talk to him? Would he go to school?* The questions were endless.

We were told by the audiologist that certain appointments would be scheduled in the coming weeks for hearing aids as part of the process, but it was quite clear that Sunny was unlikely to respond to the hearing aids, given the profound nature of his hearing loss.

Over the next weeks and months, we were called into the hospital for further appointments and Sunny was finally given hearing aids to try. He showed no progress with the hearing aids and it became clear that cochlear implants were going to be the only solution. However, as parents, we were willing to go to any length to find a more natural approach to our child's hearing loss, one that would not involve surgery and would allow our child to have perfect hearing.

We took a flight to India to find alternative therapies and treatments. We particularly wanted to explore Ayurveda - an ancient medical practice dating back five thousand years that uses a concoction of herbs to treat various diseases and conditions. We spent three months in India consulting practitioners of this ancient tradition of healing. What became clear was that while Ayurveda was quite powerful and potent in treating most lifestyle-related disorders, effective interventions for deafness were only to be found in modern medical science. With nothing further to explore, we took the flight back to New Zealand to begin the process of getting cochlear implants for Sunny.

Back in Auckland we found a local Auditory Verbal programme called The Hearing House. It specialised in helping deaf children hear and speak using cochlear implants. The team virtually hand-held us through the entire assessment process. Several meetings were arranged with families who had gone through the process already. Nothing gave us more confidence than speaking with kids as young as four or five who were talking and responding to questions just like any other hearing child. It's hard to put in words the emotions I felt after meeting the 'cochlear families'. I remember asking this one child his name and the little one being engrossed in the game he was playing; without looking up, he quipped,

"You can ask my mum and she will tell you my name!"

I was overwhelmed, not so much by the child's funny response but rather knowing that my child would be able to speak just as confidently as this little boy one day.

I felt grateful that my child was born here in New Zealand. I felt grateful that we picked up his hearing loss within a month after birth. I felt grateful for everything. To this day, my husband and I sometimes discuss that we would not have picked up Sunny's hearing loss for at least two years if he had been born in India since hospitals had no newborn screening.

In the weeks that followed, Sunny had tests and scans to determine the health of his auditory nerve before the surgery. A meeting with our surgeon, Dr Neeff, was arranged, who sat down and talked to us in a manner that made us so comfortable and so sure that we were in good hands. Sunny was about eleven months old and the doctor felt confident that Sunny would be able to handle the surgery.

On the day of the surgery, we made our way to Gillies Hospital and after a brief meeting with the surgeon and the anaesthetist, Sunny was taken to the operating theatre. A good four or five hours later, the surgery concluded. The surgeon met with us again on his way out and we were relieved to learn from him that everything had gone well. We were allowed to take Sunny home the next day.

We were probably more anxious on the day of the switch-on than we had ever been. I couldn't wait for the moment when Sunny would hear my voice for the first time. *How would he react to sound and, more importantly, how would he react to me calling him?* We were about to know. The wait was nerve-racking. The audiologist got me seated in a chair with Sunny in my arms. The external processors were fitted behind the ears on both sides of his head and beeping sounds were played to test his reaction. Sunny starting turning his head to the beeps. I was ecstatic. I had probably not experienced this kind of joy since Sunny's birth. It was an unforgettable moment as he turned his head towards me when I called out his name. I was over the moon. We were both very emotional, but this time these were tears of joy.

In the years that followed, we would visit The Hearing House once every week for Sunny's Auditory Verbal Therapy sessions. The weekly sessions went on for three years post-surgery. Lydia and Estelle were our therapists. The therapy sessions were critical to helping us parents develop the understanding of the different stages of language development and what we needed to work on at home with Sunny to help him develop listening and speech skills.

For us, the most important takeaway from the therapy sessions was that children with CIs do not automatically develop strong speech and listening skills. Close one-to-one interaction with the child during all waking hours was critical for a CI-child to develop good language. We decided one of us needed to stay at home with Sunny. We were new migrants to New Zealand and it was really difficult in those early days to run our family on a single income. However, it was something that needed to be done. We needed to put Sunny first.

I decided to stay home with our son with a singular focus – to help him not just catch up on the one year he had lost with no sound, but to work with him to the best of my ability so his speech could be as good as any other child with normal hearing. Practicing Ling sounds and making fun events out of simple chores like washing dishes were some of the ways in which I tried to keep Sunny engaged. Of all the activities we did together, Sunny most enjoyed reading with me. He would make me read twenty or more books every day and, while it used to get very exhausting at the time, looking back it was probably the single most important activity that we did together from the perspective of Sunny's language and speech development.

As I write this today, Sunny is ten years old. He speaks with complete clarity. His listening is good unless there is background noise. He is going to a mainstream school and doing well in his classes. He enjoys swimming, playing cricket and table tennis, and riding his bicycle. He still loves to read and is extremely possessive about his books. Everything Sunny has been able to achieve would not have been possible without the guidance and help of our therapists Estelle and Lydia and for this, we shall forever be grateful.

We moved back to India when Sunny was just about four. Recently we were invited by Cochlear India to share our journey with other CI families. It was our first experience addressing a large audience comprising children and families on the same journey that we went through not too long back.

Before I end this, on behalf of myself and Raj, I wish to say that we have been very fortunate. Right through our journey thus far, we have received so much kindness from people and we know we can never pay it back. But we only hope that we have an opportunity to share our learnings with families who may be starting their journey and that is why we are sharing Sunny's story.

## *Editor's Note*

When compiling this book, I chose not to add my own observations to many of the families' stories but for this little girl, I need to make an exception. I had twenty years' experience with Auditory Verbal Therapy, including having my own deaf son, when I met this family. For the first time I felt totally out of my depth when faced with advising the family what Mya's outcome would be. I had never worked with a child with no nerves visible on the MRI and with additional challenges to boot. I wondered if I should advise them to sign and forget about trying to get a spoken outcome… but Mum knew better. She was an amazing advocate for Mya from day one, reassuring me that she just wanted the best I could give, and it was her decision to take the spoken route and her responsibility. And, boy, did Mel and Jono give it their everything. I have been so incredibly privileged to work with them and see what positive parenting can achieve against all the odds! This is the story not only of an amazing little girl but of amazing parental determination and advocacy.

**~ Estelle Gerrett**

---

## *Mya's story*

# Who's in C.H.A.R.G.E ?

My beautiful moment and most positive memory of my little girl's first year was when Mum and I were playing with Mya on the floor and putting a blanket over her to play peek-a-boo. We were tickling up her legs and tummy when she let out the biggest hearty giggle. It was a really beautiful moment; Mum and I looked at each other and just burst into tears. It was the most beautiful sound I ever heard and after that, I always tried to make her laugh because she has a wonderful infectious giggle. It is still a very special memory for me. It seems such a tiny thing to many parents but, for us, it was a huge milestone and an indication that really brought me hope that my little girl could have a happy life.

The first taste of our parenthood journey was an early miscarriage just after our wedding. Which was really sad. We were pregnant again soon. It was an easy pregnancy; all was going to plan and we went for our 20-week scan. We were called back for further scans because something was not quite right. It was hard to understand because they couldn't give us a definite answer about the ways our baby looked different. I don't know if I chose to stick my head in the sand at this point and just enjoy my pregnancy or whether I was just in denial, but I watched my baby grow and felt blissfully happy. We had a lot of new things going on in our lives, a move to Whitianga, a new business and a pregnancy which were all exciting, if a little daunting. We were both still working when Mya was due. When I was ten days overdue, we decided to go out fishing, but it was not to be. As I hopped into the shower my waters broke.

We travelled to Thames Hospital and were sent immediately to the bigger hospital at Waikato. It was a harrowing two-day labour and eventually I had to have an emergency caesarean. When she arrived, they took her to the table, and I could hear a lot of muffled chatter but still did not know what was going on.

I kept asking, "Is she all right?"

There seemed to be a little bit of mayhem and confusion from the staff if I am honest, and no one was telling us much. I was a mess too and had to have several blood transfusions and wasn't really with it... I didn't even ask for my baby! Jono stayed with Mya and finally when I did get to cuddle her, I noticed she looked a little different, but I was a first-time mum and didn't really know what a baby's face should be like when first born. It was a whole lot of firsts for us both. I did notice that her ears were a little strange, her breathing was raspy, and she went very, very red when she cried. She wasn't able to feed from me, she was tube-fed my milk and I noticed that even when she was really upset her facial expression didn't change at all. So, we knew there was something wrong but still no one was telling us anything! Later they blindsided us with so many technical terms it was overwhelming, and we understood so little. We did gather that her ears were not well formed, she might be deaf, she had bilateral facial paralysis, was fed through a tube, and had breathing issues but still we had no informative conversations about Mya's future. It was just so much to take in!

Then one day when Jono was at work, the consultant sat me down alone and showed me a textbook full of pictures of children with C.H.A.R.G.E syndrome. There were no tissues in the room, and I was just completely overwhelmed. Some of the photos were just so incredibly sad of children with severe CHARGE symptoms. I just couldn't take it in. *Was this my Mya?*

Over the next eight weeks my little girl had five surgeries to release her airways and help her breathe and swallow. She went through more in her short life than I had in the whole of mine. It was heartbreaking.

Eight weeks on, I was allowed to bring my baby home. Now I was the mum of a baby with so many challenges and no support from the NICU nurses anymore. Jono had to go back to work as he had already taken weeks off to support us both and we needed the business to work. It was a really tough transition, but we just wanted to be home with our baby. I had to come to terms with the reality of a baby with multiple disabilities not just one. I had to do my very best to give my little girl a chance to be the best she could be. This first year was a year for me to learn acceptance. I really had to 'grow balls' and fight for my girl. Her ears were malformed both inside and out, with no semicircular canals and we were told she may not ever be able to walk or hear.

There were so many unknowns. We just didn't know if she would ever meet her milestones. We knew she was deaf, but it was so hard to know if she heard anything at all as she had no facial expressions to let us know if she had heard even the loudest of sounds. We tried every sort of hearing aid but we saw no response and everything was so hard to keep on her head. I felt I was batting my head against the wall. Eventually we were told they would explore the possibility of a cochlear implant. When she was nine months old, we had the MRI. It was clear that Mya had no auditory nerve on her left side. On the right no nerve was visible but they felt there might be some nerve fibres as her brain showed response to some loud sound. We didn't know if there was any hope of her hearing even after the surgery.

During this year I also began to discover that some professionals didn't like some of my parenting strategies. I was told not to put Mya in a jolly jumper (baby bouncer), but she loved it and I felt she could feel the ground under her feet and it helped strengthen her legs. I wanted so much for her to be able to be mobile. Soon she was trying to pull herself up on the furniture. As our journey developed, we began to realize we knew what was best for our girl and only listened to professionals who listened to us.

When Mya was one year old, I finally got the guts to take her out. I took her to Mainly Music and we had been going for about a month when one of the older ladies asked, "When did you find out she has Down's Syndrome?"

This hit me hard - not the reference to Down's but that someone could be as heartless as to comment on a small child's differences. It took me years to get over people's attitudes to how Mya looked and behaved. How they would stare at her or look away. This set me back a bit until I realized this was my issue really and I needed to steel myself and defend my little girl. I became quite a feisty mum from this point on. I was super protective and spoke out if anyone tried to put her in a box suggesting she was not 'quite there'.

This was the year she received her cochlear implant and started Auditory Verbal Therapy at The Hearing House. The switch-on was amazing; she heard her singing bear for the first time, and she was clacking a bunch of keys around the audiology room. Sadly, she developed an infection in the surgery site and was back in hospital for a week with the possibility that the CI would need to be explanted. I just wanted to take her home again and so asked the nurses to teach me how to administer her amoxicillin by injection and I did that for the next several weeks. We were lucky it all healed, and we could use the device again.

The following year when Mya was almost two was a year of learning for me and for her. I had learnt to accept who Mya was and I was eager to help other people to understand how much she had to offer. I also needed to get some normality back into our lives for all the family's sake. I enrolled her in daycare just down the road and Mya went there from eighteen months old until she was six years old and started school. It was new to them to have a little girl who was not mobile, but they accommodated her so very well. She developed so much socially in this year and made friends with the children she would later go to primary school with. It was such a beautiful thing to watch the other children accepting Mya for who she was.

Once again there was an incident with another adult who underestimated Mya. I arrived at daycare and all the other children had gone on an excursion for the day but they had excluded Mya! I was beyond furious and demanded to know why… "Was it too hard, was that it?". I would have gone along to help with her, if they only had asked. That was the last time that Mya was not included in anything, I made sure of that! It is so easy for others to underestimate our children with challenges. I hope that I helped that lady to think again. In many ways we were very lucky to have Mya at this daycare; it allowed her to develop and evolve at her own pace.

Mya's second year was opening up now that she could hear. It was a slow journey to start with, but we knew she was beginning to understand. This was her year to really develop under Auditory Verbal Therapy. Mya had a really cool connection with her therapist, Estelle. Mya would enter

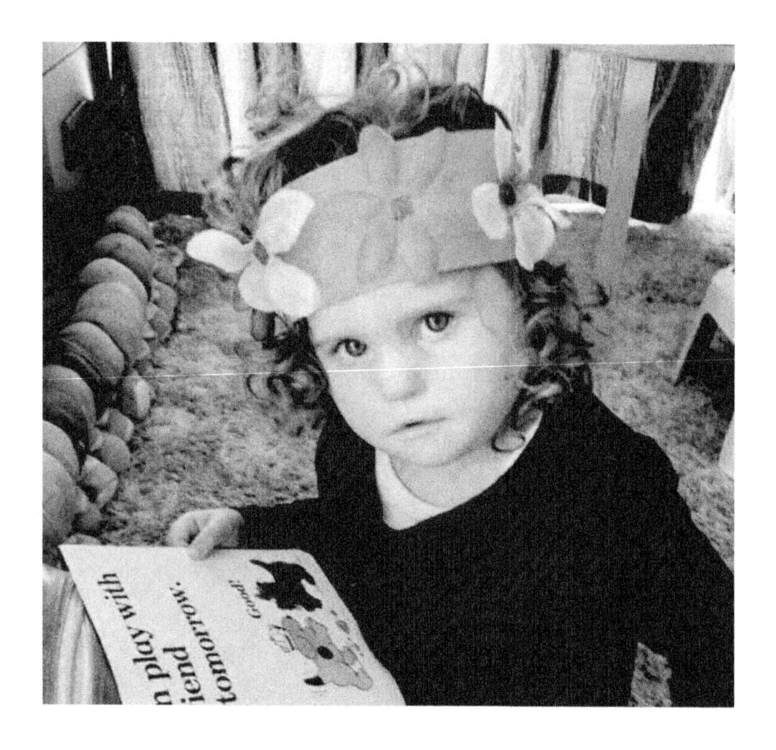

The Hearing House shouting at the top of her voice, "Stell, Stell, Stell!". She thought she owned the place. Everyone knew when Mya was in the House.

As Mya's speech developed, we had a few amusing moments as well as challenging ones. Mya had a loud voice and would often shout out when a truck passed, "Look, truck!" but since she couldn't yet produce the 'tr' sound it was substituted with an 'f'. Certainly turned some heads.

This same year Mya became a big sister to Emmy (Emerson). She was just thrilled and such a caring big sister. I couldn't get over how quickly Emmy's milestones just flew past in comparison.

There was another very beautiful moment which stays in my memory from this year. One Friday night, we were having a glass of wine and entertaining Emmy in the jolly jumper by jumping up and down with her when suddenly we were aware of Mya standing next to us! She had just stood up and walked to us unaided! We couldn't believe it! Up until then she was getting around on her knees and pulling herself up. My little girl was walking when the professionals had told me she never would. I just couldn't take it in. I rang Mum and Dad and said, "Bring champagne!".

When they arrived Mya was just walking around as if she had done it all her life! Gosh, we celebrated that night... we laughed, we cried, we hugged - it was just the best moment! It's just amazing what our brains can do. Mya was three years old when she took her first steps. Now our girl does cross country with all her peers.

Mya loves hospitals and loves appointments and has a real confidence visiting. She is such a positive little girl. By the time she was six, Mya had attended a lot of appointments in hospital and some of those were with a plastic surgeon. Mya has bilateral facial paralysis, which means she can't smile, can't close her eyes, or control her nasal fluids. We had the option of smile surgery which would entail two major surgeries in which a muscle would be removed from Mya's inner thigh and inserted in her face near the location of the facial nerve. It was a very long operation and quite an ordeal to connect all her vessels to ensure the face could move. Her surgery did work, but not as well as hoped. It certainly helped with her speech clarity though as she could move her mouth more.

Now at six years old, Mya is at a small rural school in the village. We are still having a few toileting issues as she doesn't have the same sensory feedback from her bladder as most of us do. She needs to tell herself to go to the toilet as part of her routine. Her first teacher was quite stern and harsh, but it seemed to help Mya learn structures and routines. I did have a few issues with this teacher getting frustrated with Mya. I knew this because when she had toilet accidents at home, Mya often said, "Don't tell teacher, she'll be mad at me". I asked for her teacher aide to support this at break time, which really seemed to help her read her body cues.

Mya loves reading and thrives on it at school. She has always loved books and reading but writing is a challenge to her motor coordination. Just learning to hold the pencil took a lot of effort. Her motor coordination is still a challenge, but she gives everything a go; dodgeball, athletics, cross country - she always gives it her best shot. I love that about our school: everyone always gives her the best shoutout when she finishes. It is a very inclusive little school and supportive of everything she tries. We are lucky to have a lot of help and support both financially and educationally from the local authority to adapt the school to Mya's needs. Now these adaptations are used for other children who have mobility challenges too, which is cool. As a mum, I still worry that

Mya has no real friends, but I think that's just my perception. She is happy in herself and loves to go to the library to read when it's break time. It is maybe something that will change as she matures socially. Listening and speaking have allowed Mya a rich and full life in a hearing world.

As I write this, Mya is speaking to the whole school on Book Day to thank her librarian for all the help she has received. She is excited and confident to speak from the stage!

---

*If you have a child with additional challenges, the journey is a marathon not a sprint. Don't rush the milestones. Savour each achievement and enjoy the successes and keep your eyes on the prize. Remember you are strong enough and you are not alone... You can do this!*

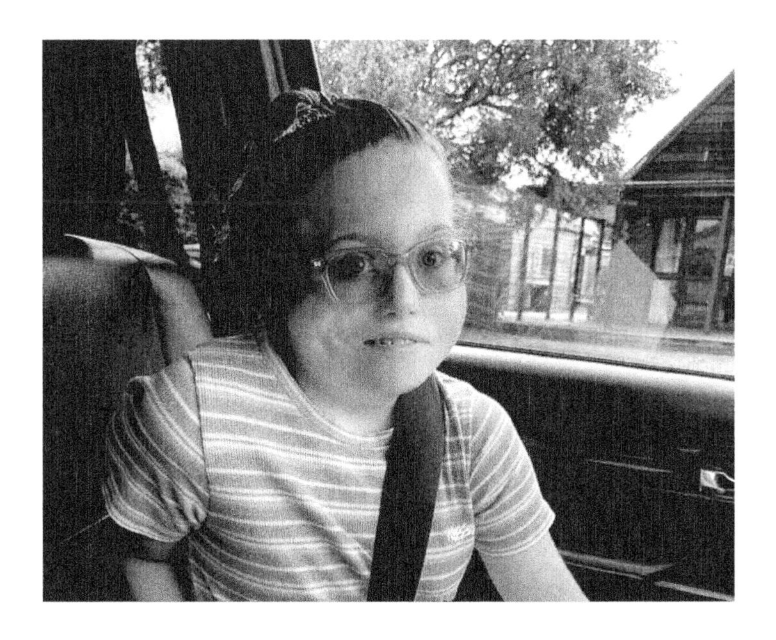

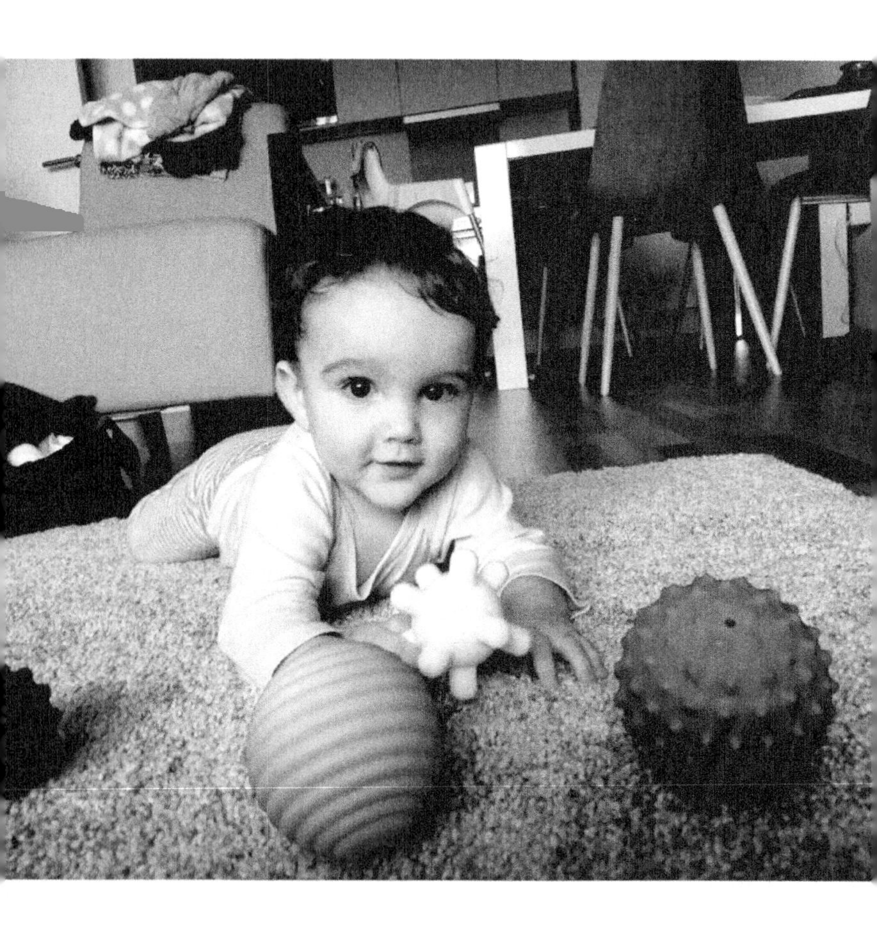

*João's story*

# Love, faith & family

## OUR BILINGUAL JOURNEY

Here we are again. While the UK is mourning the late Queen Elizabeth II, we are at the Great Ormond Street Hospital for another long three hours of waiting. It is his third time; our son João was implanted in October 2018, and due to a manufacturer's recall, he was required to explant both sides and reimplant again.

We had been here before to replace the left side just earlier this year. As we left him behind in that cold room yet again to replace his right side, my wife and I started to reflect on our journey so far and what kind of learnings we have had along the way since we learnt about João's condition.

João was born on 1st November 2015, in São Paulo, Brazil. He passed his hearing test in the maternity hospital, so we believe João had hearing for some time at the beginning. He was slow to talk and was babbling his first word, Mama, at about one year and five months old. He was diagnosed with severe/profound sensorineural hearing loss on 31st October 2017, just one day before his second birthday. The Great Ormond Street Hospital assessment and surgery list together took another eleven months of João's time. He was implanted for the first time on 5th October 2018.

He started Auditory Verbal Therapy at AVUK in April

2019, graduating from there in June 2021. We always worked in Portuguese as this is his mother tongue and it was important that we were giving him the richest language possible as he started his journey to speech. We worked alongside Estelle, an English-speaking therapist and translated everything for João and worked on the goals in Portuguese at home. As his understanding began to develop, we also paired his learning with English as he would need this in school. He still does Speech and Language Therapy twice a week privately to help him master the new language concepts and refine his speech clarity as he was implanted late.

Overall, it has been a tough journey full of learning and rewarding moments. This is a journey where you get completely detached from what you once knew was a standard and start to see and feel the world completely differently.

It was in 2018 when we joined this rollercoaster journey full of anxiety, fear and unanswered questions. In the middle of all these, we followed three simple but powerful principles that drove us forward and made us see things differently and face the upcoming challenges.

The first principle is **Family**. We could crumble as a family and each one of us follow our own path and João would be lost in the middle of our grief and our individual weakness. Instead, we chose to face it as a couple relying on and supporting each other and developing stronger foundations for our family. This enabled us to face everything we have conquered with him.

The second principle is **Love**. It drives us forward, from the way we do things for him, the devotion and dedication to his education, his rehabilitation and empowering him to live a normal life. This is reflected in the way we adapted our lifestyle to accommodate his needs, allowing us to dream big. All we have done, and all the journey we have had so far is based on unconditional love. Without love, it would have been impossible to move forward and overcome the challenges we had. The relationship we have with our little one today evolves as the love grows, it is visceral and heavily based on touch and feel more than words. I can't even imagine how our life would be if it was not for him, or how our life would be if he was not deaf. We love our son the way he is and his uniqueness, and we never regretted or resented it for one single moment. We are pleased to have him - he is our most valuable gift. A divine gift.

This leads us to the third principle, our **Faith**. Without our faith, nothing would be possible. Faith is the fuel that kept us going and keeps us moving forward. We are a faithful Roman Catholic family, and we do not just create João into these values, they provide most of the unanswered questions in our prayers. We have lost count of how many nights we spent awake crying and praying for his future once we learned he had "bilateral severe sensorineural hearing loss", also known as Deaf. The inspiration of a bright future and the strength we extract from this faith are as key as the love that moves us.

God was and is still very much present in our lives and is always helping our family to overcome everyday challenges. And today it is no different. João is now in his hands while the doctors replace his implant and we patiently wait, anxious but trusting that God has him in his care.

As part of this journey, we also met some special people, people who in a very unexpected way inspired and taught us about a completely new universe. One of these unexpected friends is James King and his mother. He didn't just teach us a lot about this new universe of deafness and the challenges we would face after João's implantation, but his mother gave us one of the most valuable lessons back in 2018 when we met both for a family lunch. On that occasion, we were facing the complex National Health Service (NHS) assessment to identify if João would be eligible to receive cochlear implants. As a family, we were living through the grief process and Vanessa left her career behind to look after our 'poor' deaf child. I still remember the face James's mother made when she asked if João was at school, and we answered that he would stay at home with Vanessa until he gets implanted. She looked at our eyes and said,

"Never treat João as a 'poor' child. He is healthy, smart and happy and he is no different from the other kids his age. I never treated my son with pity, and you know how far he has gone."

After that lunch, Vanessa and I changed our perception, she restarted her career and João started nursery.

João has just started Year 3 in a mainstream school and he is bilingual (Portuguese and English). He still has gaps in his communication, but we are now confident that he will close these gaps soon. His English is catching up with his Portuguese really fast. He loves music and sports. He plays football (as a keeper) every Saturday and practices Taekwondo twice a week, enjoying his life with his hearing peers.

We just got the call we were waiting for, and João is back from the surgery room and waking up from the anaesthetic. All went well and soon the right side will be up and running again.

The biggest takeaway from our story is that our future and the future of our children is shaped by the choices we make every day, regardless of whether they have a special condition or not. As parents, we have a responsibility to support them to succeed and make sure they have all the necessary devices to do so. The number of hours dedicated to his speech-language therapy, and the investment we made in surrounding him with the right professionals is paying back and I have lost count of how many times I asked him to be quiet for a minute so I can hear my thoughts. Such a wonderful feeling to ask your deaf child to be quiet, so very normal.

All this dedication is worth it because it is based on the three principles we mentioned before. We hope by writing this that it will help someone to see the challenges they may have ahead with different eyes and face those challenges with hope and positivity. If not, I hope I made you smile with our story.

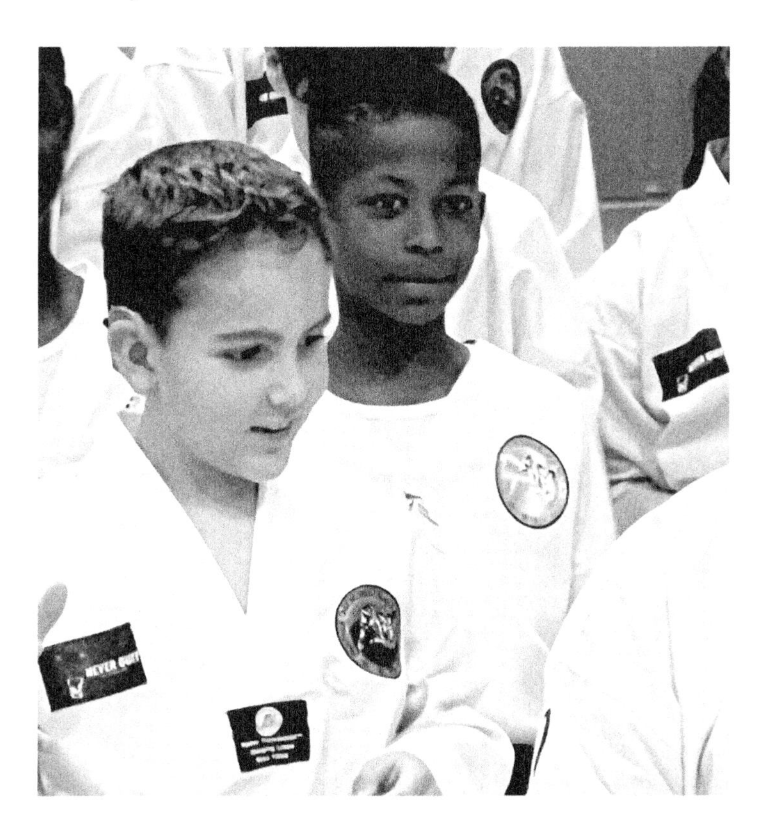

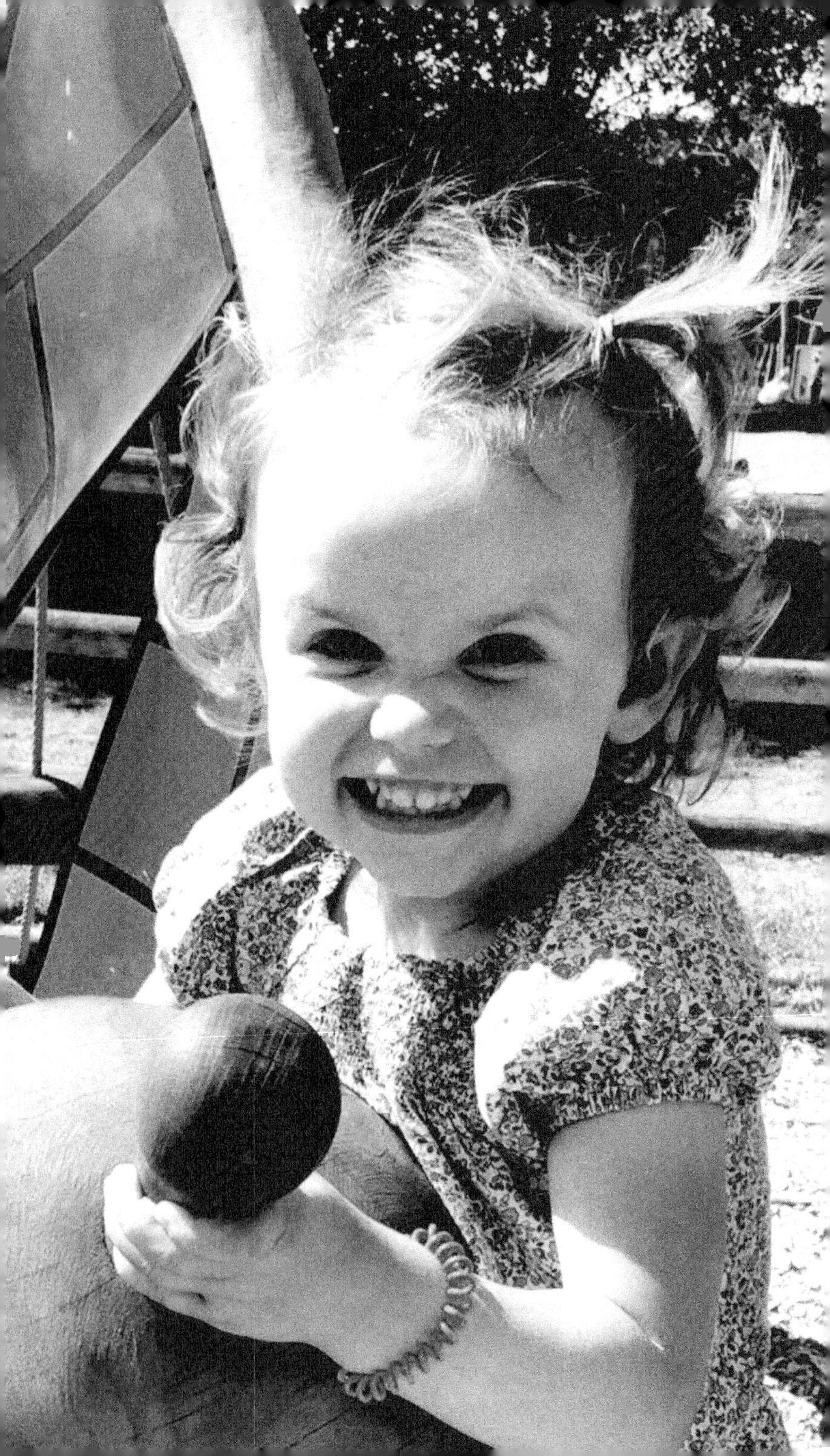

## *Prudence's story*

# A mother's guilt

The guilt, the mother's guilt, the mother's guilt mixed with the guilt of a teacher of Special Educational Needs who should know what she's doing. I should be an expert.

I can still hear the thud now. The thud of my baby daughter's head on the newly-tiled floor and her crying, crying so hard that she is holding her breath and turning blue. The cries of a frustrated, angry baby who is not being understood by her family, the ones who love and know her. The ones who should be able to look at her and be in tune with her needs. Me, looking at my husband, James. James is the fixer in our family, he's the one with all the answers and here we both are, asking each other, "What do we do?". And in the panic, looking down and seeing our other little girl at only four, looking up at her sister with a puzzled look but learning to accept that this is the new normal for our family.

What had happened? We thought we had it all. I was a successful teacher working three days a week and James was working extremely hard to start up and run his own business. We had not long bought our house for our family of three when we discovered we were expecting again.

When we discovered we were pregnant, we were thrilled at the thought of expanding our family. We already had Fleur who was coming up to two years old when we discovered this. Being an only child myself and seeing how close friends of mine were to their siblings, I was excited for the adventures they would have together.

Fast forward nine months and there I was having the waterbirth in our local birthing suite that I had longed for the first time round. We were now parents to two girls and our newest addition was named Prudence and she slotted into our family life like a dream. Prudence passed all her newborn checks including her hearing test. Like her daddy, she was loud and wild. When she entered a room, everyone noticed Prudy. We were a busy family, with endless baby groups booked and regulars at our local play café. (Little did I know that this would become my therapy.) The weekend would come and you wouldn't see us for dust; we loved a jammed-packed lifestyle.

I remember sitting wrapping presents the night before Prudence's first birthday, thinking, *Where has that year gone?!* However, I can't remember much else because what was to come in the next year would somehow erase the happy memories of her first year. (I hadn't realised that until right this moment of putting pen to paper!) Anyway, her first birthday I do remember and sadly for the wrong reasons. It was a sunny day in spring, and we had family coming over throughout the day to give Prudy their birthday wishes but she wasn't her usual self. She was grumpy and at times quite distressed and no matter how much attention she received and how many cuddles she was given, she wouldn't settle. I put it down to it being a busy day and that she may be overtired (tiredness being my reasoning for anything and everything when the girls were not on top form).

Prudence reaching the milestone of being a year old would also mark me returning to work after maternity leave and continuing the juggle of being a part-time teacher alongside being a mummy. I moaned about trying to have it all but when I look back now, gosh, I loved it! Loved being part of a team, feeling valued and knowing that I was making a difference to the young lives of children who had their challenges. Little knowing that the real challenges of my life were just beginning...

Now we were hitting the summer and James had suggested taking Fleur away for a week, just the two of them, before she started school. Two days in, I rang him.

"Prudence isn't responding to her name, but don't worry, it's probably glue ear. Glue ear is so common with young children," I said to him. However, by the end of their week away I was calling him again.

"James, it's not just her name. She isn't responding to anything."

At this point I still wasn't concerned; I had always thought we had been so lucky in life so far and that the luck would continue. Like I said, James is the fixer and with the stretched National Health Service system, he wasn't prepared to wait. So, on James' return we contacted The Portland Hospital, where all the celebrities that I read about have their babies. I was intrigued to go and see what The Portland experience would involve.

The day came and there we were with Prudence having her hearing check and the audiologist was performing the tests. He stood behind her with a drum the size of the old-fashioned bin lid. He banged the drum, no response, banged it again, no response. Why I wasn't concerned at this point, I do not know. I think I was naïve. In my head I was thinking, *I have brought my daughter here because I believe she has glue ear, and I am waiting for you to confirm she has glue ear. What do we do next?* Then he said the words that I won't ever forget:

"She could very well have glue ear, but I just have a feeling there may be more to this."

Even after him saying those words, I STILL believed she was going to get a glue ear diagnosis. An hour later, she got the diagnosis that we had come for and we were to await her operation date for the glue ear to be drained and her grommets inserted. The operation came and went, and it had all gone to plan.

Then all the messages from friends came:

"What is she like after the op?"...

"Is she able to hear you all now?"

The answer was no; no, she couldn't but we had been warned this may be the case. From then on, things started to unravel; November 2019 came and we went back for the post-op hearing check. Still very little response but there was some flicker of hope. We went back again, and we were told that "those with a large build up in their ears can take longer to recover."

Then January, February came, and we were back in London again for her final hearing check. Still not much of a response. Slowly it was beginning to trickle into my head that something may be a little amiss with regards to her hearing. We were sat there, and James' phone was going bonkers with work calls, and he popped out to see what was going on. Nothing much was happening in the test room; they were going through different procedures. Then the lady said,

"She's very young but she seems bright. I am going to try a split ear hearing test. This isn't something we usually do with children so young, but we'll give it a go."

Then the lady turned to me. "I'm very sorry but Prudence is profoundly deaf in her right ear and has moderate to severe loss in the other. I know this must be such a shock."

Yes, she was right, it was a shock but at least now we had an answer and an answer with a solution: hearing aids.

She repeated, "This must be a shock, it's okay to be upset," and then I found the tears trickling down my face, Prudence smiling away and playing with all the noisy toys, the noisy toys that she could barely hear. And at that moment in walked James. He looked over to see me crying, "What's happened, what's the matter?"

By this point, I couldn't share the news, I was just too upset. He was told and soon we left. On the way home, I could tell James was devastated that he wasn't there by my side as the news landed, but how was he to know? I certainly didn't feel any upset that he wasn't there, but I know for James this was a big deal. He wants to be present for everything which involves our girls.

I can't remember much more from that day.

The evening of 16th March came, and our Prime Minister Boris Johnson announced a national COVID-19 lockdown. I was already having a much-needed Easter break from work and at school we had discussed having an extended holiday of maybe two more weeks. What a ridiculous thought when you look back now.

Then life for our family erupted. Now, this may seem less like a recount and more like just a series of episodes because if I am honest, I don't remember much, other than how awful it was being stuck in a worldwide pandemic with a child who required medical attention.

So here are some of Prudy's episodes...

Prudence is bright, no doubt about it - she has her daddy's brains for sure! But with that came huge frustration when unable to communicate her thoughts within a hearing family.

Huge frustration looked like this for Prudy...

Banging her head on a tiled or wooden floor whilst hysterically crying and if we attempted to pick her up, she would throw herself backwards.

Crying so much that she wouldn't be able to catch her breath and she would then turn herself blue. I still couldn't tell you what the cause of some of these moments were, or what she was trying to communicate. I would just hold her tight and rock her, backwards and forwards, side to side.

She made herself projectile vomit to show that she didn't want to do something. She liked to make this move when not wanting to go in the pram or at bedtime. I can semi-laugh about it now because those days are over but, bloody hell, it was bleak, especially as we couldn't ask family for help because of the lockdown. The days seemed so, so long.

Then came the biting stage. I found this even more upsetting because it was Fleur who became the target for these outbursts. Prudence bit her, which made Fleur bruise, and she would pull handfuls of Fleur's hair out too. Again, I can't tell you the cause but for the most part it was when Fleur received any sort of attention from me. We were attempting to home-school Fleur because of lockdown. I deliberately use the word 'attempting' because I am not sure what Fleur learnt during this time as our homelife was so turbulent.

I do remember one day Fleur sitting online, camera on, ready to attend her virtual lesson. Prudence was insistent that she should be part of the lesson, however she wouldn't let Fleur appear on the screen too. I leant over and nudged the camera towards Fleur so that she could see the learning taking place and then Prudence dived in and bit Fleur hard. Prudence screamed and Fleur burst into tears, followed by me. I knew this was happening in our home before but now it was being shared with the class and the class teacher. That made everything even harder for us all.

YES! Schools were back open - but that set a new list

of challenges. I could never predict when Prudence was going to have one of these moments and I used to pray that she wouldn't have one whilst trying to get Fleur ready for school or on the way to school. I didn't want others to see our struggles.

Then the acute guilt came again. All the mummies at school knew of my position at work and yet they were witnessing daily my lack of ability to manage my own daughter's behaviour and needs. I remember one mummy seeing me scoop Prudence up off the carpark where she was having a moment to 'express' herself. I wanted the ground to swallow me up and to just hide and have a big cry. I felt like my reactions at times reflected on my ability to do my job... When it is your own child, it is VERY different.

In amongst all of this, we had received a diagnosis that both Prudence and I had tested positive for Cytomegalovirus. I had everyone being supportive with comments like "You mustn't feel guilty", but the truth is, I didn't feel guilty. Why would I feel guilty for something I had no control over and that I had no idea I had? I did however feel deep sadness. Sadness that something that I had contracted would now change the life of not just Prudence but our whole family.

I lose track of time scales, but we were sneaked in between various lockdowns and fitted with hearing aids. This gave some relief to the frustrations Prudy was facing daily but not enough to make a huge difference. However, I do feel having some access to sound albeit very little did give her some comfort.

Then we started meeting with Estelle from Auditory Verbal UK. This would consist of listening therapy sessions for Prudence which either happened over Zoom or, when the pandemic allowed, face to face in London. Prudence's diagnosis was still new to us, and it was comforting knowing that Estelle had a child with hearing loss and could empathise with the guilt of trying to juggle Prudy and her sister. Prudence was making some progress, but it was slow. Then there came a time when I was finding it more and more upsetting because her hearing loss was deteriorating due to the CMV and the sessions were becoming trickier for her to access.

Estelle asked me, "What would you like to do going forward?"

It was the first time Estelle had ever asked us this before so deep down I knew that Estelle was aware that Prudence's access to sound was very limited and that this was hindering her Auditory Verbal Therapy sessions, but Estelle knew it was important for us to come to that decision ourselves; we needed to be the ones in control. It was at this point we needed a break and waited for a date for cochlear implant surgery. Estelle promised to still be on the other end of the phone if we needed her, and we promised to tell her when we received the phone call for Prudence's operation to be implanted. She had been on the journey with us so far and was keen to see it to through to the end.

So, then we played the painful waiting game. The waiting game of hoping your child will become 'deaf enough' to qualify for the NHS criteria for cochlear implants. I don't think James and I even discussed the pros and cons of the operation, to us it was our only hope. YES! She was finally deaf enough! The best advice we had been given by Estelle was to be a polite nuisance and to call weekly to ask where in the lineup we were. That job was given to James, he is far better at those tasks than I am.

Due to COVID, the timetable of implant operations was reduced but we did get told that they were keen to implant children before they were three years old, and we only had a couple of months before Prudence was due to turn three. We will be forever grateful to Anna who led Prudence's case at Southampton University Hospital. We felt confident that if anyone was to get Prudence to the top of the list it would be Anna. It's all a blur but I think we got THE phone call on the Monday and then on the Thursday she was in for her operation. I can remember crying down the phone to Anna, I couldn't believe this day had finally come. I can imagine for many families they would feel worried about the operation but despite being one of life's biggest worriers, I didn't. I think what I felt was relief, relief that Prudy would finally be able to hear; this was going to be the answer to the last two years of hell for our family.

Then the 4th of March came - operation day. Only one of us could go into the hospital because of COVID restrictions. James having the gift of the gab when needed sweet-talked the man at the door and got in so that he could be there for Prudence to be registered and admitted. James then had to leave, and I accompanied her to the ward. We were so fortunate that we had our own room. When we got the nod, Prudence was wheeled down to theatre and the life changing day would begin.

After three hours we returned to hospital, me to the ward and James to the car to wait. We wouldn't see each other for the rest of the day but it didn't sit right with him to go home whilst Prudence was still in theatre. The operation was far longer than we were told and took double the time and some! Finally, the nurse came in and told me I could go down to recovery. Estelle had also given me two questions to ask the surgeons. The first was to ask if they had inserted a full array (all the electrodes of the device) and secondly if the NRT (neural response telemetry) test had shown positive results. This would inform us whether the operation was a success. Estelle also told us don't be alarmed if she bleeds from the mouth. Top tips that really helped to calm me on the day.

The next day Prudence was discharged with her medicines and off we went.

After a few weeks of recovery, she was fit and healthy enough for switch-on. Now, I had seen all the Facebook videos of children having their 'ears' fitted and them looking around in wonder at the new world opened. For Prudence,it certainly didn't look like that and, having spoken to other parents of hearing-impaired children, it didn't for them either. Obviously a lot of social media hype. Instead, she refused to wear them, and this would start a new set of frustrations. I don't know how many times I cried that week, cried to the hospital, cried to anyone who would listen. Then we took drastic action. James took a day off work, and we tackled it the three of us (the three being James, myself and the biggest bag of chocolate buttons known to man). I think that week 90% of Prudence's diet consisted of chocolate!

Months went by and we resumed our therapy with AVUK. Prudence was a happy cochlear implant wearer, and she began to show glimmers of the Prudy we knew pre-hearing loss. We had started a little bit of sign alongside spoken language as at times noise levels were loud and I needed to be able to communicate with her. I knew that she had taught herself to be a visual learner.

I knew Prudence was making progress with her spoken language but having nothing to compare it to was killing the teacher inside me as I wanted to measure her progress. So, when asking our teacher of the deaf about how well she was doing, she said to me, "Larah, you have got eight months before she starts school. If there is any way that you can afford to maybe stop work for a little bit to support her at home, I think she would benefit from your skills and being in a language-rich home environment."

Juggling work and being a mummy to a child with additional needs as well as a mummy to a hearing child who needed to feel her mummy's love more than ever was becoming too much. James and I made the decision that I would step away from my career. It didn't sit right with me that I was enabling the children in my class to progress but not allowing my own child that opportunity.

Christmas of 2021 came, and I hung up my lanyard after working at my school for fifteen years. My days would now consist of being at home.

They say that, after a storm, comes a rainbow and that's how I would describe the next months that followed. For us, the implants had been a success and Prudy was beginning to fly. It started off with naming objects and then a couple of words together at times, a mix of sign and a mix of words. She was really coming on and family members were noticing.

Then someone mentioned The Elizabeth Foundation in Portsmouth. They opened their doors and arms to us as a family and Prudence started in the February. There was a class of about seven children, and she would attend once a week. Prudence would scream with delight when I told her it was a Rachel and Emma day. She felt at home there and, with that, her confidence grew and grew. They had a two-way mirror in the room so that parents could stand and watch their children in action. Or in my case, stand and watch whilst trying to stop myself from crying at all the children's progress.

All the parents together became so invested in the progress of not just their own child but also each other's. It sounds cheesy but it had that 'one big happy family' feeling. It would also become my weekly therapy as I struck up a friendship with a mummy from Prudence's class whose son also had CMV, and we would chat about our experiences. I sobbed and sobbed when summer came, and Prudence could no longer attend as she was now to start mainstream school.

School was a daunting thought; we were unsure if she was ready. We looked at mainstream schools and schools with a resourced provision within the school for children with hearing loss. When looking at schools it became clear which schools were willing to take on a challenge and which were not with comments like, "Well, we can't offer her any quiet space within the school". As I was being told this, we were stood in the school's library with one child doing exactly that, working in a quiet space. Other comments included, "It will be far too noisy for her at lunchtimes". *That was fine,* I would think, *I don't want you to have her at your school anyway,* and off I would trot.

The Elizabeth Foundation was right, she was ready and, as I write this, she has been at school for nine weeks now and guess what... she flipping well loves it! We chose a school which has a resourced provision. We chose a school who said they would be stretching her strengths as well as supporting her weaknesses. She has a group of friends, she's had play dates with friends, school discos, you name it, she has thrown herself into school life. We've recently had parents evening when they shared with us that, at the moment, she is 'on track' for her maths, writing and reading abilities. We couldn't have wished for a better start to her education. I'm sure it's not going to all be plain sailing but for now we can take a moment of feeling proud.

Nothing fills me with as much pride as when I look at Fleur and her relationship with her sister now. At times, it can't have been easy for either of them. I hope in years to come when they are both grown up and making their own ways in life that they both look back and think 'our parents did the best they could during a tricky time' and that they realise any decisions we made, we only ever had their best interests at heart. We will always do all that we can to enable them to achieve.

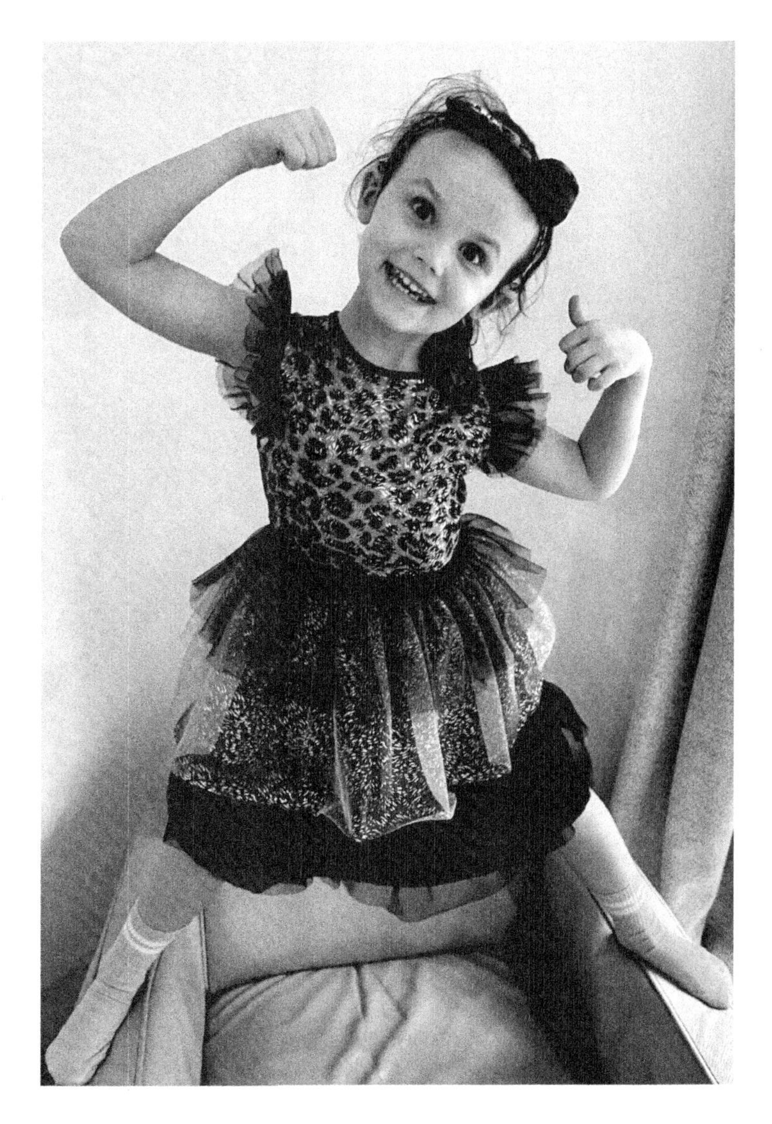

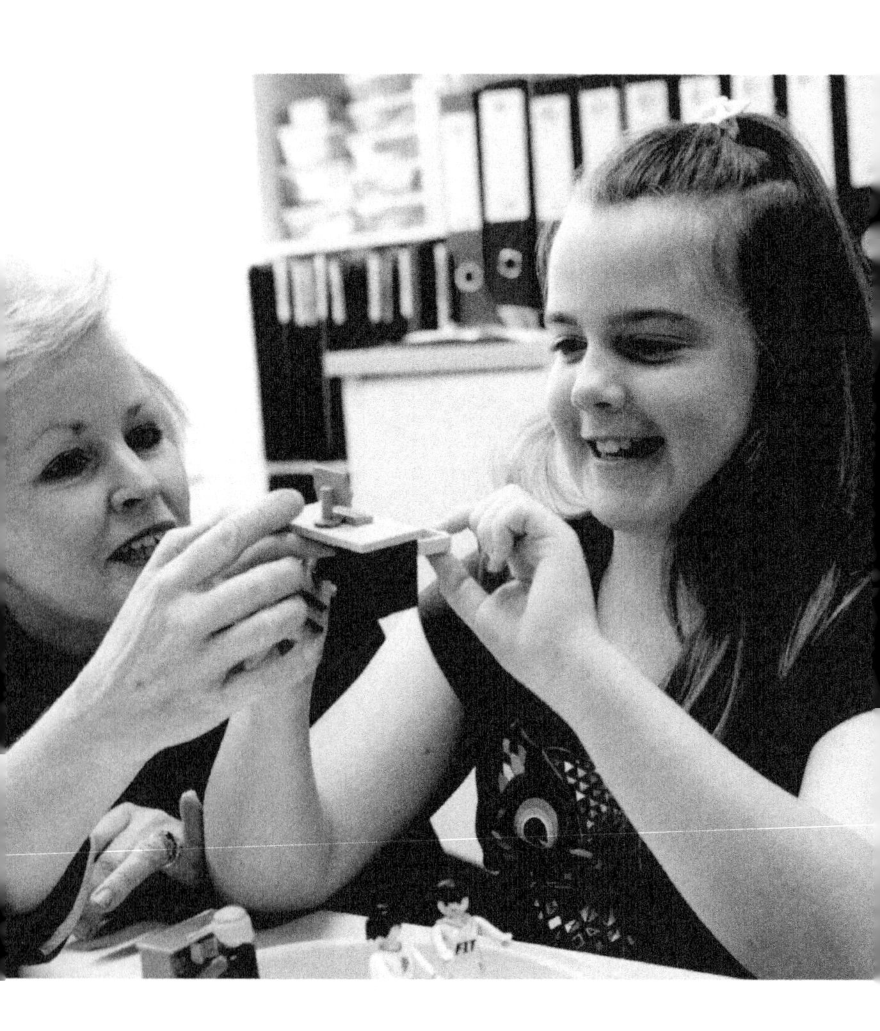

## *Tahlia's story*

# Wow! Wow! Wow!

As I read through what I have just written, the hearing journey of my girl from complete silence for the first two and a half years to a non-stop talking young woman, I am overwhelmed with so many emotions! What a journey we have been on and writing this shows me how far Tahlia has come. From the beginning when we feared the unknown and many sad tears were shed to where we are now, so extremely proud of her and crying tears of happiness. Wow! Wow! Wow!

On 1st August 2004, Tahlia Abbie came into this world to join our family. She was welcomed into our very excited household by her big sister Kaylee, who was twelve at the time, big brother Jacob, who was nine, Mum and Dad and of course lots of extended family.

When Tahlia was about nine months old, I was concerned that she was silent apart from crying. She didn't babble and hadn't said the words we all wait with anticipation for: "Mama" or "Dada". My other kids had talked quite early but with comments from others like, "She has her siblings to talk for her" or "She'll talk when she wants to", I convinced myself it would happen in her own time. But deep down I knew something wasn't right. She was achieving all the other childhood milestones at the right time, if not before. She wasn't a sickly child. She had never had an ear infection, not even a cold. Finally, after several visits to the doctor over a period of six months, I asked for a referral to have her hearing tested at Starship Hospital where shortly afterwards we were told our little poppet was profoundly deaf in both ears. Wow! The last year suddenly all made sense. This was the reason for the strange but funny things Tahlia would do or the uncontrollable behaviour. My constantly having to run after her because she wouldn't stop and having to keep my eyes on her all the time so she wouldn't hurt herself because she wouldn't listen. She COULDN'T! She was in her own little world, not knowing any different.

For me to hear the audiologist say Tahlia was deaf was a huge relief. Now we had an answer. It was a starting point. After three months (from referral to the appointment), many different diagnoses had run through my head. Family and friends were great, with awesome support and love. I sometimes felt I needed a tape recording when answering everyone's questions but I know it was all out of concern, love and interest, and I greatly appreciated it. Our immediate family just carried on as best we could, speaking normally to Tahlia and including her in everything we did. She made up with her eyes what she couldn't hear and we filled her with lots of different experiences and sights. Kaylee and Jacob were fantastic. We just kept telling them Tahlia was exactly the same as she was before we knew she was deaf. They compensated beautifully, always making sure Tahlia could see their faces and making sure she could understand. An awesome big brother and sister! You could read Tahlia by her facial expressions and gestures. And she was very good at them!

Tahlia was diagnosed as having Auditory Neuropathy. Her ears were working fine but the nerve which takes the sound from the ear to the brain was damaged. We were told that she probably would be a good candidate for a cochlear implant but there were no guarantees because of the auditory neuropathy. From there, we began an assessment programme which over six weeks involved many appointments at Starship, a visit to a paediatrician, a psychologist, a CT scan and the beginning of our wonderful journey with The Hearing House. Tahlia also tried out these gorgeous tiny hearing aids for six weeks but they didn't help her at all. At the end of the assessment, it was decided that Tahlia might benefit from a cochlear implant. We were elated! We had an opportunity to give our baby the gift of sound.

On 28th January 2007, Tahlia (now two and a half years old) had her operation at Gillies Hospital to insert the internal part of the implant. At the time Tahlia received her implant, they only funded one so she was implanted on her right side. It was nerve-racking but very exciting. She recovered quickly and bounced back to her cheeky little self within a couple of days. On 7th February 2007, armed with a video camera to capture the moment and our hearts full of hope, we arrived at Greenlane Audiology. It was time for the implant to be turned on. Tahlia heard sound for the first time in her two and half years of life. Truly, truly a miracle! She was fine for a few minutes, pottering around and then she became very frightened and began to cry a very sad cry. My heart broke for her. It was very overwhelming. With the encouragement from the CI team, we took her home with very quiet footsteps and voices to start a brand new way of life. A new beginning.

For the first two weeks, I felt like a horrible mum. When it came time in the morning to put the implant on, she would run away and protest with lots of tears. Finally when I would get the implant on and switch it on, she would sit still like a statue for about fifteen minutes, very upset, only moving her eyes as if afraid to move. I had thoughts like *What have I done?* but I knew I had to do it. She gradually became used to it and soon learned to put the implant back on herself. She would come running if it came off while playing. She even went to sleep with it on as she didn't like to have it off at all, in case she missed out on something, which was great! There were many more visits to the Greenlane clinic for the adjusting of her map, gradually bringing her hearing level up to normal volume. But it was so worth it!

I dealt with public perception of Tahlia's behaviour often. Mostly the behaviour or her very loud demanding was out of pure frustration at not being understood. We would have a lot of loud meltdowns. She knew what she meant and wanted, it just took us a little longer to work it out.

For example, a member of the public in a shop came up to me to let me know that my daughter sounded like little dogs fighting and I shouldn't let her make that noise - while I was just so happy that she was making any attempt to communicate. I had to learn to ignore what other people would say or think and tried to keep my mouth shut, which could sometimes be very hard. Usually, I would just fiddle with the implant and people would slowly move away, very embarrassed. I didn't need to say a thing!

The next step in our journey was to teach Tahlia how to listen and speak. This is where the wonderful Hearing House and their very patient staff came in. We were made to feel very welcome, and it was very much a safe haven for Tahlia and me. I now had contact with other people, staff and parents who were travelling the same journey as we were, which was incredible and so freeing in knowing that we were not alone. We began our Auditory Verbal Therapy journey with weekly sessions and were always made to feel very welcome. As the primary caregiver, I would attend these sessions and bring the activities, poems and songs home where we could all as a family continue to work on the week's goal.

During Tahlia's time at The Hearing House, we had three therapists, Liz, Lydia and, as she neared school age, we moved on to work with Estelle. Our family are so eternally grateful for the patience, support, confidence and kindness shown towards Tahlia and myself by these three wonderful ladies.

Progress with Tahlia over these first few years was slow and steady. Her receptive language was great. She learnt several words, to come when her name was called (which was amazing!), and she could follow instructions, but her speech was our hardest hurdle. Just before Tahlia started school I was told that maybe because of the auditory neuropathy the implant wasn't doing its job quite as well or that she may have apraxia of speech, which is when someone has trouble saying what they want to correctly and consistently. This was really hard to hear and comprehend, but we battled on.

As Tahlia graduated from The Hearing House, Estelle found us an awesome private articulation specialist, Liz Fairgray. Tahlia started going to weekly speech therapy sessions and her speech improved. She worked with Liz for two years from the age of five to seven. These two years were very much a turning point in Tahlia's speech and you could see the changes in her. Her speech became so much clearer, conversations with her were starting to happen and she learned to stop and think about what she wanted to say before she said it, slowing down the process. It was as if a lightbulb had gone on and something had clicked! It was an unforgettable experience to watch my little girl who had struggled for so long now start to communicate to the world, to be heard and understood.

Tahlia attended The Hearing House Preschool at the age of three to five and a half. The preschool was a community preschool, which children both with and without hearing loss attended, and it was based next to The Hearing House. The preschool teachers were given the information from each therapy session and told what we were working on that week, and they added it into to the play activities Tahlia was doing at preschool. She absolutely loved it and the staff were amazing with her and very patient. Many hours travelled, three times a week in peak hour traffic on an Auckland motorway from the North Shore to Greenlane for kindy, but worth every centimetre!

I decided not to start Tahlia at school until she was five years and eight months old as her speech was still very much delayed, so she continued on at the preschool, had extra sessions at The Hearing House and speech therapy with Liz.

When the time came for Tahlia to start school, I was so nervous and unsure of what her future might hold. It was scary! *Would she fit in? Would she have friends? Would she be able to keep up with her peers?* She was the first and only child to have a cochlear implant at the school, but they were very willing to learn about it and what Tahlia's needs would be. It all turned out to be an easy transition for Tahlia and the staff were excellent. She had ORS funding, which provided her with a teacher aide for class time and she had a resource teacher of the deaf who visited twice a week. Within a few months she was well and truly settled. She made friends and she was on a level with, if not above, her peers in all subjects.

That first year of school saw a big improvement in her speech, going from a two-word phrase to speaking in full sentences. Amazing! Her 'tantrums' due to lack of being able to converse with her peers or get her words out correctly continued but with patience and consistency and Tahlia's ever-growing speech, they started to diminish. She used an FM system consistently at school, which was a great help. She can tell you a few staffroom conversations as well, when her teacher or her teacher aide forgot to turn it off at breaktime! Tahlia was also given a time-out-from-the-classroom card, which she would show the teacher when she needed a bit of quiet, as a loud noisy classroom could sometimes be very overwhelming for her - too many different sounds and tones all at once and very tiring. Individual Education Plans were also a new experience but a vital part of Tahlia's education. The SENCO, class teacher, teacher aide, the RToD and myself attended the IEP meetings and worked together to put a plan in place for Tahlia to succeed at school with the supports that she needed.

Tahlia continued to flourish throughout primary school both speech-wise and academically. She was so lucky to be able to have the same amazing teacher aide throughout her time at primary. Mrs Walker advocated for Tahlia all the time. She was there for her both academically and emotionally, and stood up for Tahlia when I wasn't there. For that I will be forever grateful. Tahlia found a love for sport and played netball and basketball and competed in Rippa Rugby. She also started to play softball for the Northcote Softball Club. She never let her hearing loss stop her from doing anything, something I am extremely proud of her for. Her stubbornness was now paying off!

Through school, Tahlia also did drama and ballroom dancing with Johnny from Dancing with the Stars. That was Tahlia! Always wanting to try something new and be involved.

During this time Tahlia started going to the Kelston

Deaf Education Centre (KDEC) sports days in Henderson with other deaf children aged from five to eighteen years old. They were a day off school with Lynne, her teacher of the deaf, and she absolutely loved them. Kids just like her! Lynne also got Tahlia interested in the speech competition in Hamilton, which is a yearly event where students from all over the North Island read a speech they have written. They are judged by a local high school principal and teacher. Tahlia loved this as it was a chance for her to meet up with friends she had made at previous events. Lynne was a huge help and a true blessing while navigating Primary and eventually the transition to Intermediate.

In 2014, when Tahlia was in Year 6, we were given an amazing opportunity with the generous help of both sets of grandparents to gift Tahlia a second implant. She had been wearing a hearing aid in her left ear every day, not for sound but to keep the hearing nerve active for when she could have a second implant and have two 'ears', as she called them. We were warned and told once again there were no guarantees: because of the auditory neuropathy, the second implant may not have much effect or any effect at all, but it would give her more spatial awareness (the ability to distinguish where a sound came from) and as a family we wanted to give our girl every chance. So, in December 2014 we headed back to Gillies for the operation. A week later it was switch-on, and a very different experience to the first time. She could let us know what she was hearing because this time she knew how to talk and could describe what she was hearing and how she was feeling. Estelle visited us during the Christmas holidays and helped us with listening exercises and advice on how to strengthen her new 'ear'. Tahlia worked very hard at home and school to learn how to listen through her new implant until both ears sounded 'normal' and 'equal'.

When it came to which intermediate school Tahlia was to attend, we chose not to go with our local but to send her to another where only a handful of students from her primary would be going. We talked about the choice together and decided this would be a fresh start and somewhere she was not known as 'the deaf kid'. It was the best decision we made! Her teachers and the staff were amazing. She went from having a couple of friends to making lots! She thrived. She loved learning and did amazingly well while still adjusting and learning to listen with her new implant. Academically she was still equal or above her peers. Literacy was her favourite subject with her love for writing and reading.

Her passion for drama was born and she was in two school performances, The Lion King and The Wizard of Oz. She continued playing netball, basketball and softball. Lynne, her RToD, also kept her involved with the KDEC speech competition where she placed third. In Year 8, Michelle became her new RToD and continued to provide tremendous support to Tahlia and the staff.

It was so incredible to watch my beautiful, strong, brave girl embrace everything she could and overcome the difficulties her hearing loss gave her while trying to achieve and give the best she could. On the day I received the news my little girl was profoundly deaf in both ears, there was no way I would have ever thought these things possible.

In 2018, Tahlia started at Birkenhead College (Secondary School) and the teenage years began. Her love for learning continued. In late 2017, before her college years commenced, Michelle, Tahlia and I held a meeting with the Year 9 dean, deputy principal and learning support teacher to discuss and agree on Tahlia's needs, such as how the FM worked, where she should be seated in the class, having subtitles on all videos, etc. One of the things we discussed was that we didn't want Tahlia to learn another language. It had taken eleven years to get her to this stage of listening and speaking English! The school were supportive of this and instead timetabled a period of Learning Support in the learning centre run by a wonderful teacher, Mrs Coker. The learning centre provided a much quieter environment with just two to four students in there at a time, all doing their own class work with help there if needed. Tahlia also had some yellow cards which she could show to any teacher. These enabled her to leave the classroom and go to the learning centre to continue on with her work in quiet. We all remember those college classrooms, don't we?! They can be very loud, boisterous and distracting! And listening, especially focused listening, can be exhausting for our CI kids. Mrs Coker was also involved with Tahlia's IEP meetings and was a great promoter and advocate for Tahlia with the other staff when sometimes she would need to remind them that Tahlia was deaf and they needed to face the class while talking, not face the board, or have class notes written down and available to Tahlia, which she desperately needed with six different teachers in a day, all with different accents!

All of these preparations and considerations for Tahlia starting college were great for my peace of mind as I felt the same nervousness I had when my little girl first started school. Tahlia, being Tahlia, took everything in her stride with her head held high and walked in on her first day ready to conquer whatever lay ahead and made many lifelong friends.

She became a great ambassador for overcoming the obstacles of hearing loss. She could now self-advocate and took responsibility for her own learning and achievements. So proud!

We had a new teacher of the deaf start with us, Anna, who

again helped so much with the transition between schools. She worked with Tahlia for almost a year before we had our old friend Michelle returned to us. She invited Tahlia to talk to a conference of teachers from schools around the North Shore about what it was like to be a deaf student in a classroom, and what the teachers could do to make school a better experience for them. Tahlia loved being an advocate for herself and the deaf community and given any chance to do so, she did. She wanted people to know that she could do anything anyone else could do and her hearing loss didn't stop her!

Over her time in college, Tahlia achieved and grew so much, and made some lifelong friends. She received many certificates of excellence in all subjects, but the most rewarding thing has been the compliments that I have received about Tahlia. Her confidence and perseverance have shone through. She absolutely LOVED her time at college! It gave her so many opportunities and she took them all. She once again competed in the speech competition in Year 9 where she placed 2nd; Year 10 she placed 1st and in Year 11 she took the highest award, the Most Extraordinary Speech and Topic Award, and received a huge trophy! In Year 10, Tahlia also entered a speech competition through mainstream school competing against students from other schools. She was the only one entered from her school and she placed second. My child, my deaf child who took so long to produce clear and understandable speech, was now delivering winning speeches! Unbelievable to me!

Tahlia has spoken in assemblies to promote topics around deafness, such as Sign Language Week and Loud Shirt Day. She has been a community leader and was on the Arts Council. Tahlia loves the arts. This came through in her subject choices, which included drama, art, photography, and art design. With drama, she took part in two school productions, Monty Python's Spamalot and Puffs, which is a take on Harry Potter. In Puffs, she had a main character with speaking lines!

Tahlia still continued with sports, playing for team 2 in netball and U19 girls basketball. In Year 13, she decided to take up football and she still plays softball. She was part of the North Harbour Softball U15 girls team and travelled to Palmerston North to compete in a New Zealand-wide tournament and is now playing in the club's top team for women.

In Year 11, Tahlia was awarded 'The Dean's Award for Year 11' for Overall Excellence in Year 11. I sat in the audience and watched with my heart bursting as my girl - my girl who was born profoundly deaf, who didn't start to talk properly until the age of seven, who had overcome a lot of ups and downs in her hearing journey and worked so hard to get to where she was - received the top award for her year level. The look of surprise, happiness and pride on her face when her name was announced is something I will always remember.

In that same year, Tahlia was also nominated for and won the Deaf Children of New Zealand Makero Mason Cup for Excellence in Year 11, which is a nationwide award. Deaf or hard of hearing students are nominated and need to have two or more letters of recommendation from their school. She received another huge trophy and $250!

And to finally end the most unbelievable year, she was asked to be on a youth panel at 'Listen Up!', a National Federation for Deaf and Hard of Hearing conference. It was held at Sky City in Auckland City and Hillary Barry was the MC. So, Tahlia and I dressed up all flash and fancy and headed off, not quite knowing what the day would hold but, as always, any chance Tahlia could get to speak and advocate for the deaf/hard of hearing, she would take it on 100%! The aim of the conference was to enlighten employers on the hiring of deaf people. It was an amazing day for her to be a part of.

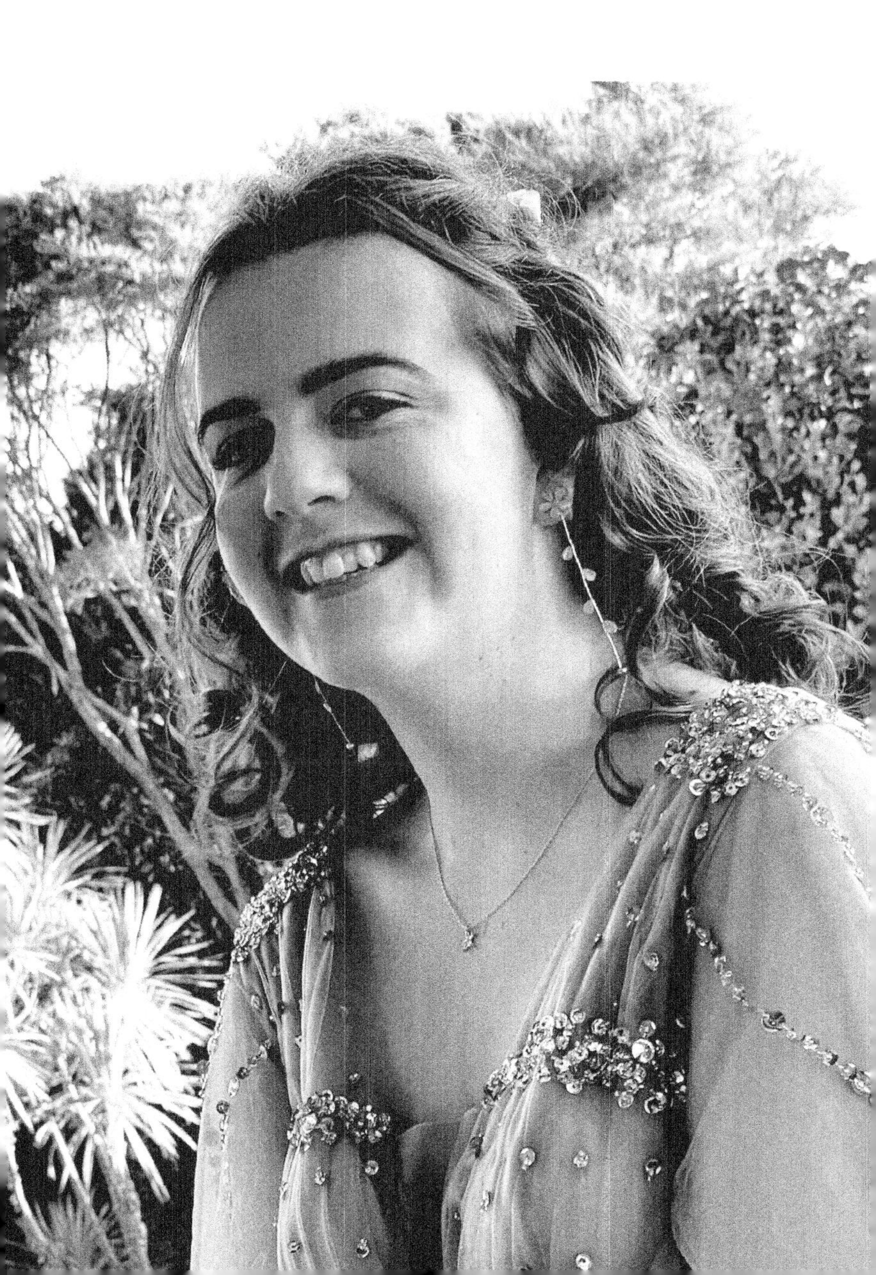

And then COVID hit our beautiful country and all schooling went online. Tahlia did miss out on the school ball, which of course was cancelled, and many other fun things, but she kept up her social contact with friends through screens and carried on with school work. School work was actually better online than in person for some subjects such as English and History where there was a lot of teacher talking and writing notes. Having these provided online worked out better for Tahlia. Zooms were okay for her as the teachers were great at the mute button! And she often had one-on-one Zoom meetings with her different teachers.

Returning to school after many months of lockdown and now with the use of masks was difficult for Tahlia and I'm sure most of our deaf and hard of hearing kiddos. Tahlia is still only 70% hearing when wearing both implants so still relies a lot on lip-reading, which you cannot do when everyone is wearing a mask! Her FM system became even more important and it was used a lot more. The school was great and her friends really understood how hard it was for her and were very patient and accommodating to her needs. Everyone worked with Tahlia on what she needed and we managed the best we could. And she finally got to go to her first and only school ball.

Everything started to go back to normal after COVID, just with a few more rules, and in 2022 Tahlia completed her final year of college.

Halfway through the year, Tahlia and Hannah discussed her options for university. Hannah then organised a trip to both Auckland University and Auckland University of Technology (AUT) to have a look around and talk with the disability help there to find out what was available for Tahlia such as a reader/writer and scholarships for the hard of hearing. Hannah then organised help for Tahlia with her transition to university through Geneva Health as Tahlia will be moving out of the school system and will no longer have a teacher of the deaf.

In October 2022, Tahlia applied to both Auckland University and AUT in the city to do a conjoint Bachelor of Arts degree, English and Criminology and Criminal Defence with the goal of becoming a lawyer one day. And she got into both! She has decided to go to AUT as a few friends are also attending there and Tahlia likes the facilities they offer for their students with hearing loss.

And that is Tahlia's journey so far. A long and windy, sometimes very bumpy journey but it has been one of the best and one of the hardest journeys our family have been on. We have in no way travelled this journey alone. We are privileged to have been blessed with the most amazing therapists, teachers, teacher aide, resource teachers of the deaf, family, friends, coaches and team mates on this journey with us and their patience, kindness, love, support, help, advice, care and interest shown to Tahlia have helped shape this confident young lady who manages her hearing loss so well and is able to listen and speak with purpose. There is no way to express how thankful I am and how much I appreciate their impact on Tahlia's life.

And now we wait with so much pride, excitement and anticipation to see what Tahlia's future will look like and what it holds for her but no matter what the outcome, I know she will always be the awesome, brave, strong, funny, kind, feisty, confident person she is.

Wow! Wow! Wow!

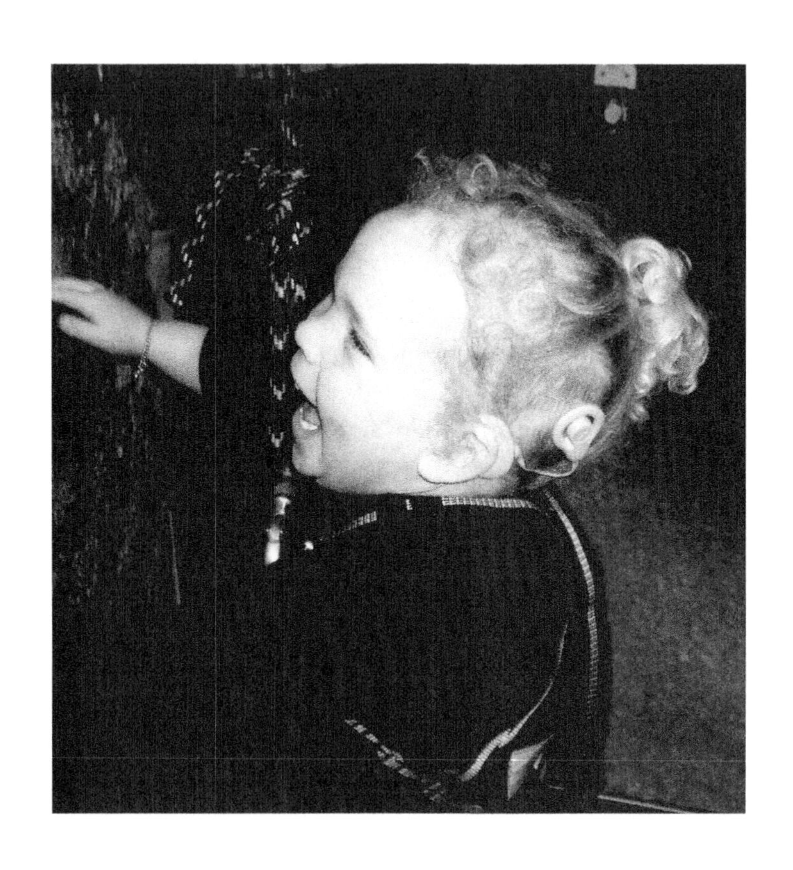

## *Elly's story*

# A life-changing illness

July was always a holiday month for our family and this year was no different even with three sick children, two having chicken pox (post infectious) and our youngest with rotavirus. After doctors had cleared them all okay to travel, we headed off to Auckland Airport for our flight to Christchurch, then a short drive to Hamner Springs for a winter holiday with great hot pools close by. Once we arrived, just one stop to get supplies from the supermarket for the week and let the fun begin... at least this was the plan!

Just twenty-four hours in and Elly, now nearly fifteen months old, was showing signs of illness. All she wanted to do was sleep, sleep, sleep so we put her in the pram and set off out to get some fresh air and play putt-putt golf with the older children. Elly wasn't enjoying the outdoors or the brightness so kept herself snuggled up in her blanket. At this point we both thought it was just a typical childhood illness.

Upon return to our unit, we rang the doctor as Elly was not keen to eat or drink. The doctor on duty was busy so they sent an ambulance. While waiting for the ambulance to arrive, the doctor came and cancelled the ambulance. He checked Elly out and decided she was dehydrated and needed fluids so tried to put an IV line in to start the rehydration process. After trying both her arms and feet, he still could not get a line in as her system had started to shut down. She was vomiting and almost unconscious by this stage. Pete and I knew this wasn't just dehydration, it was something more, but the doctor kept trying to get a line in. The frustration was great as I wanted her to be checked out at the hospital, but the doctor wasn't keen. Finally, he did call the ambulance back and rang through to Christchurch Hospital for advice. When the ambulance came to collect us, we were told to keep trying to give her water in her sipper cup for the journey.

On arrival at Christchurch Hospital, we went straight into a cubicle and the doctors began to check Elly out. Shortly after we arrived, two doctors and two nurses were with her, and she was reacting to the light and the fact they were trying to take all her clothes off. I thought this was a normal reaction for a child in a strange place, late at night with strangers hovering over her. One doctor picked up that she was light-sensitive and next minute they wheeled her away and into a special room away from us. They suggested to us that she may have meningitis and they were going to do a lumber puncture to test. We were freaking out. Our other two children aged five and six years old were put into an isolation area because of their chicken pox even though they were no longer contagious. My husband and I waited in another room. This was the most heart-wrenching time. We couldn't all be together and support each other and emotions were running high. We were all alone and so were our children. We had to trust the medical professionals around us even though we didn't even get to meet them first as it was all hands on deck with Elly. It was really hard.

What seemed an age later, the doctor appeared to advise us that Elly had pneumococcal meningitis, stating she could die in the next two hours, and we needed to be prepared. They were administering five different drugs to help her fight the disease. Now we needed to decide who would go in the helicopter with her to Starship Hospital if need be. What a decision! One of us would be left behind with two children and a long journey back together, and the other would be alone with Elly possibly when she passed. Not a decision to make lightly. Not easy for either of us.

Time passed and it felt like hours and hours, but it wasn't in reality - it just felt that way. Elly was transferred to a High Dependency Unit. She was so pale and lifeless that she looked like she had passed already but the monitor told us otherwise.

As much as I didn't want to be alone with Elly, I didn't want to not be with her either. Peter drove back and packed up while I stayed and tried to rest, keeping one eye open watching Elly's machine beeping. Twice during the night her alarms went off. Her body temperature had dropped so low that they had to tuck her into a heated blanket, warming her one degree per hour. The first twenty-four hours would be live or die, then the following twenty-four hours would reveal how well she would come out of it. There was a possibility of deafness, blindness, seizures, organ damage or any combination of these.

Once we were out of the painful forty-eight-hour window, Elly's chances of survival were better. Two days later, she was responding well to the drugs, getting a little colour and wanting to sit up. Elly spent four long days in the HDU, then was transferred to a ward where she continued with her multiple injections. This was extremely unsettling for her as it would take two nurses to administer the medication and two nurses to hold her down so they could inject her. Elly stayed in the ward until she was able to fly back to Auckland and travel via car back to Hamilton with our family. She was given medication for the flight back and then we headed directly to Waikato Hospital to be admitted as a patient there and continue her treatment. It was a stressful, nerve-racking time for us all and panic struck when our flight was delayed. We were worried about getting back in time for her next medication. This was just another difficult point in our journey, worrying what may happen to Elly if we didn't get back in time and how she would last for the flight. Luckily for us, the delay was short. Arrival at Waikato Hospital was a relief for us all as we were on home ground and had family around to support us.

Eventually, Elly was allowed home but went back in twice a day for simultaneous injections in her thighs and doctor catchups for the next five days. It was still draining but also rewarding that she could be at home with us in a semi-normal environment during the day and spend time with her siblings and family. We knew now that she would live.

Once life was semi-normal again after about six weeks, it seemed that Elly's hearing was not as good as it used to be. We started baby sign and kept an eye on other signs of impact the meningitis may have had. Nobody had checked Elly's hearing before she was released from hospital.

Within three months of contracting meningitis, Elly had totally lost her hearing and we had started investigating options. Only one Auditory Brainstem Response procedure per month was being scheduled at Waikato Hospital. There was a waiting list and Elly was fifth on the list. We waited patiently for our turn. Finally, seven months post infection, Elly was diagnosed profoundly deaf in both ears. Tears of sadness and delight were shed as, up until this point, we had been unable to access any help or support without a diagnosis. We ourselves had known she was deaf and so used New Zealand Sign Language to help with our basic communication.

Living in a small community, we found it extremely difficult when word got out that Elly had meningitis. Her siblings, Olivia and Mitchell, were kicked out of a school carpool we had going as the other parents were scared their children would catch it. Parents at school did not talk to me but were happy to point and chat about us amongst themselves. I needed to take action!

I put together a folder with information about our journey so far and how it had impacted our lives, making it clear that our older children were not treated while Elly was in hospital, as meningitis wasn't contagious. This folder and its contents were advertised in the school newsletter and left at the school office for parents to read it if they wanted more information. Several parents asked my opinion on the vaccine and if they should vaccinate their children. I would respond, "If you have any questions, please consult your GP." This was something I did not want to comment on or be responsible for.

I do think that putting something in a school newsletter or making something similar available to your child's school is important. You can also add links or offer your email if anyone has any questions. I really think this made a difference. Some parents came and approached me saying, "I've read your booklet." We chose to include pictures of Elly as well, to help build the understanding of where we were at.

Our family was welcomed into an Auditory Verbal programme at The Hearing House where Elly qualified for a cochlear implant and so her process began. Elly received her first cochlear implant at the age of two years and one month, and so started on her journey towards being able to hear through this device. Later that year Elly's ENT, Colin, suggested it may be a good option to put a dummy implant in to her other ear to save the space from ossification as it may not be possible to give her a second implant later. We agreed as we had nothing to lose. (Cochlea ossification is one of the damaging side effects of meningitis. It means that the cochlea can go hard like concrete and if this happens the surgeon may not be able to implant. Elly's first implant surgery took longer than expected as the surgeon had to drill away more ossification than expected.)

We were lucky enough to have Estelle as our Auditory Verbal therapist whose son was also deaf from meningitis. Her understanding of meningitis was comforting along with her professional expertise.

The programme allowed us to connect with other parents in our locality and also in the Auckland region. We attended events and this also enabled Elly to make friends with other CI- and hearing-aided children.

In Hamilton where we live, we tried to get a group of parents to meet but after about a year of trying we decided it was not meant to be, due to lack of parents attending. There were other groups running in other regions that allowed us to join them for a period of time. This was a great benefit as we were able to attend camps, outings, dinners and general fun days where the children could hang out with people who understood the challenges without having to talk about them out loud. We were able to chat with other parents, most of whom we could relate to in some way, with no judging, just understanding, all with different stories.

Once Elly was well underway with her habilitation, there was a little more information coming out about the advantages of having bilateral CIs. As there was no available funding, we decided to pay for Elly to have a second implant. She was implanted at three years and two months old. The baby ear (second implant ear) only took about five months to achieve the same hearing level as her originally-implanted ear. We noticed a huge difference in her directional sound ability.

Our journey has been eventful. We've been involved with many groups, met lots of people and supported others during their initial stages to help them see some light at the end of the dark tunnel. Elly and I got involved with the Meningitis Trust and we have been at a couple of presentations to talk about our journey. A highlight for me was when we had a peaceful protest outside New Zealands's Parliament Beehive.

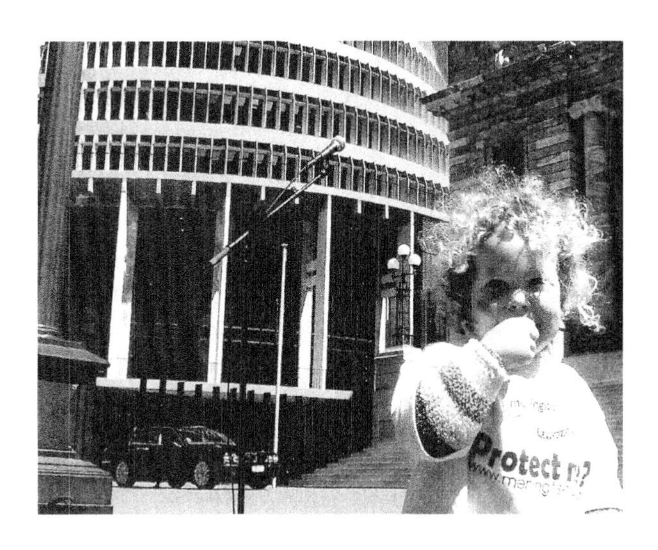

Two lucky families were asked to come inside and express their concerns around the vaccine and the funding of cochlear implants. We were one of the families that were chosen. To see the reaction on the ministers' faces when they heard the cost involved for a family to purchase a cochlear implant and pay for the surgery showed clearly what an eye-opener it was for them. New Idea magazine ran an article about Elly and her journey to bring awareness about meningitis and its long-term effects. Attitude TV came and recorded an episode at our home with our family and interviewed us as part of the Meningitis Trust as well. Elly's siblings Mitchell and Olivia took part in a fundraiser, Shave/Braid for Meningitis, and it was well supported and gave them a feeling of being able to help. I like to get the message out to everyone who's prepared to listen: THIS IS A SILENT KILLER.

We were once told it would be five to six years before we could see the damage pneumococcal meningitis had inflicted on Elly and this is a true statement. In the first year her liver was oversized and she caught every bug going, but after that she developed an amazing immunity, which she still has...so some positives too!

When she started kindergarten for a few hours a week, Elly was fortunate to get renewable funding which gave her access to a resource teacher of the deaf and also a teacher aide when she started school, for which we were very grateful. This is when were put in touch with Kelston Deaf Education, which over the years has enabled us to get resources and support at school. I joined the Board of Trustees as the Parent Representative. During my time on the Board, I was also lucky to meet, speak to and work alongside some great people and try and give as much input to Deaf Education as possible to help the children of New Zealand.

Elly has a passion for sports, and this has helped her mix and mingle with other mainstream children even though she is currently in a Physically Assisted Unit at her high school. She has taken part in a SEED programme with Countdown Supermarket for one day a week for six weeks; she did herself proud and they gave a fantastic report. During this year (2023) she has also passed her Baby-Sitting Certificate which allows her to have more independence. Over the Christmas period she has also secured a work experience job at the local doggy daycare. She had written her CV and emailed it to the owner herself, so this success was very rewarding for her. At the end of her second Year 13 at school, she has just completed her final paper for Level 1 NCEA English and has sufficient credits to pass, 54 credits at NCEA Level 2 and 22 credits at NCEA Level 3. We could not be prouder of her and are very grateful for the team she has surrounding her, who help her achieve these goals.

Mitchell and Olivia are also a great support for us as they encourage her to take part in sports, social activities and general everyday activities that keep her active and socially engaged. We are currently working on Elly gaining flatting skills as she sees herself living away from home with support and we admire this decision.

Something I have learnt from this is that *Life is precious, and you need to go with your gut feelings.* We are ever so grateful to have Elly alive and with us today. She has brought great joy to our lives along with some struggles, which have made us stronger people.

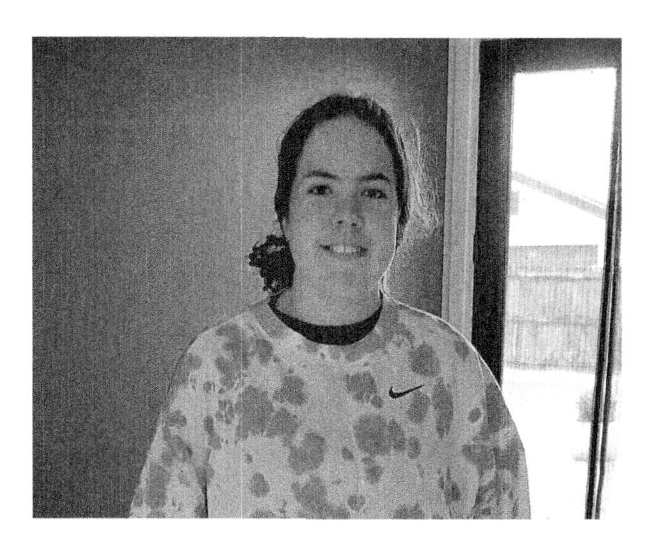

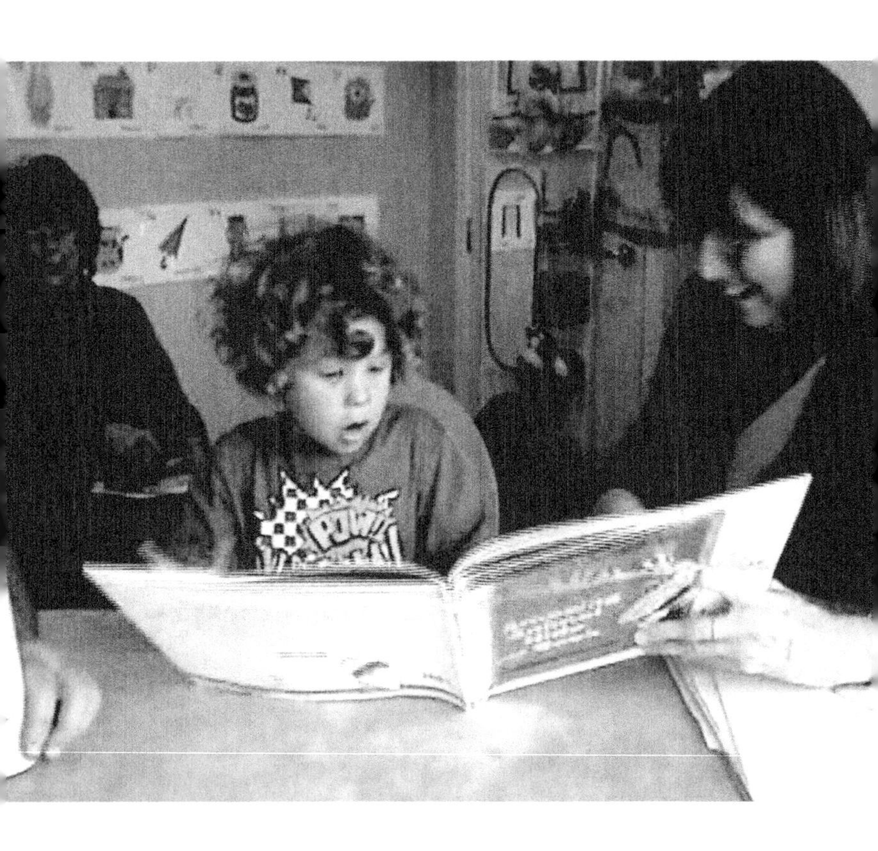

# *Ollie's story*

# Let's hear it for the boy

So, this was it. She was leaving and I was alone.

With an unrivalled sense of clarity and calm that I had not experienced before, my path forward had just smacked me in the face, and I could not have been happier. At that moment, I went from running on adrenalin and being on the brink of a breakdown to an overpowering sense of being in control with a clear direction of where I was heading. This challenge was to be mine going forward, it seemed.

My name is Gary, and I am father to a profoundly deaf child named Ollie.

The path to Ollie becoming part of the hearing and speaking world has been filled with plenty of highs and lows, laughter and tears, but it's a path I have been most fortunate to have walked with Ollie and held his hand along the way. It has been a privilege and a true learning curve for me.

Ollie was born on Waiheke Island, New Zealand. All seemed pretty normal from what we could see. He was a happy, healthy and engaging little baby boy. After a while, my mother noticed that Ollie wasn't responding to her voice and discussed it with me; I discussed it with Ollie's mother and she also said that she had noticed the same. He didn't react to any noise, you could call him or do the vacuuming, bang some pots and nothing, no response. It was clear that something was wrong.

He was taken to Auckland Starship for hearing tests but the tests proved inconclusive. It took a total of five visits and eight months before Ollie was finally given an ABR and it was discovered that he was profoundly deaf in both ears. I remember it well, being told the news and I took it very calmly. It wasn't until we were heading home that the devastating news hit me. I remember feeling numb about what I had just been told, a million things were going through my head:

*How will Ollie deal with this?*

*How will he be able to make friends?*

*What things will he not be able to do?*

*How do I deal with this?*

*What will this mean for us and how we live?*

*Will we have to shift from the island?*

*Where will we need to be located?*

*How will we communicate?*

These questions whirled around in my mind, a combination of worry and pragmatism as to what would need to be done.

One of the most important things to happen at that time was a home visit from our adviser to the deaf, Nick. I am so grateful for Nick being there at that time. Ollie was diagnosed on the Friday afternoon and Monday morning

Nick was at my home on Waiheke Island, giving us some reassurance that there was support for Ollie and giving me some solid information on our options and a way forward. It was exactly what I needed. I felt now that we would at least be able to make a plan.

Nick told us that we basically had two options for Ollie: he could attend a signing programme at Kelston Deaf Education or be assessed for a cochlear implant.

"A what?" I said.

I had no experience of deafness, no one in our family was deaf and I had never heard of an implant. Nick explained the process to me and I was really excited at the thought of Ollie being able to listen and speak. We opted to investigate the implant with a profound sense of excitement. He explained that to have a really successful outcome, we as Ollie's parents needed take responsibility for his learning - the commitment really falls on the parents to ensure a good outcome.

It wasn't long before we were being introduced to the wonderful staff at The Hearing House. It was our local Auditory Verbal programme. There was a warm and friendly feel about it, and we were made to feel at ease. We were taken through the facility and told of the procedure. It was made very clear to us that a big dedication was required from both me and Ollie's mother. We were told that Ollie would need to wear hearing aids for a period of time prior to surgery. This was to see if they would be suitable for him instead of an implant as he had a little residual hearing.

Soon after, we started our therapy sessions at The Hearing House with Alexandra. This was a baptism of fire for me, totally out of my comfort zone. Alexandra had me making all these silly noises and playing silly games. I noticed there was a camera in the room, and I was waiting for her to say, "Hey Gary, smile, you've just been on TV bloopers!". But no, this was the real deal, this is how it's done. I had no choice but to accept my plight and play along with Alexandra's ways. I learned how important it was to check Ollie's devices and use something called the Ling sounds to check he was hearing properly. Unfortunately, most of the time I was the only one attending with Ollie. I couldn't understand why. We had been given this wonderful opportunity to have our son lead a pretty normal life, but it seemed that the commitment necessary to achieve this was largely going to fall on me alone.

So here I was, looking after three kids, one of them profoundly deaf, doing most of the work at home and trying to keep my business afloat, pretty much on my own. One day we returned from therapy to find Ollie's mother lying on the couch watching TV.

"How was the therapy?" she asked.

I asked her why she wasn't there, and then asked her to leave. So now here I was, alone with the responsibility for Ollie's future and all the financial commitments too. Despite this, I was happy; happy in the knowledge that I had absolutely made the right decision for Ollie and myself. In essence, I had been doing it all alone anyway and I knew I had to get on with it.

Things picked up markedly from that point. I couldn't carry on with my work and do everything that was required for Ollie. My decisions were easy, I simply put Ollie first.

I had shares in our family-owned business, so I opted to sell them in order to reduce the mortgage on my home. At that point, my parents made an offer of help with Ollie; they took on the role of the second parent, attended therapy with me and helped me follow up on all the goals and work we were set. Our day started with Ollie and I at home doing our learning about listening, then off to creche to allow me to work. My parents would pick up Ollie in the afternoon and spend time helping and teaching him until I would pick him up after work. We soon realized that listening and learning were to become an integral part of our everyday world. All in all, things were running pretty smoothly, everyone was a lot happier and we had a clear plan of where our journey was taking us.

Ollie was a handful though; he would take great delight in smashing stuff; his favourite trick was to get the plates out of the kitchen and drop them on the floor. He thought it was hilarious when I would shake my finger at him and say "NO! That's naughty." I guess from his perspective it was great entertainment smashing stuff and having this crazy guy opening and closing his mouth and waving his hands around. He so obviously couldn't hear me although I guess my face probably said it all. He loved to run away from us, any opportunity he would take off and be delighted in the chase, laughing his head off. I remember one incident clearly when things got a bit out of hand; I couldn't find him anywhere and eventually saw eight little fingers clinging onto the edge of the window of the second storey of our home. I pulled him in. Window and door latches went on the next day.

The hearing aids were a disaster. Ollie hated them. He would pull them off all the time, LIKE ALL THE TIME. He would hide them anywhere he could. When I look back, that was the most frustrating thing as I was constantly keeping an eye on him for any sly antics. It seemed like this period would never end while we were waiting for the implant surgery. I just hoped that it wasn't going to be the same with the implants.

Ollie was soon under surgery and having his op. I felt quite at ease with Ollie having the operation although there were those normal concerns of whether this would work and allow him to hear and speak. Once Ollie went into theatre, I went for a walk to take my mind off things while keeping an ear out for my cell phone in case of a call from the hospital. Michel Neeff, Ollie's surgeon was great to deal with and he was very happy with how things went. I was not nervous at all; having great communication and being informed of what was to happen gave me total confidence in Michel. I knew Ollie was in good hands.

Switch-on day came around, with Ollie, both my parents and I waiting in anticipation of what was to come. It was a pretty anxious time, but we were rewarded with wide eyes and an exclamation from Ollie indicating that he had just heard his first sound. I was not sure at first if it was a good indication of success, but it was clear upon several more responses from Ollie that he was hearing. It was a huge moment for us, but his response was a little underwhelming and after the testing, Ollie carried on as if nothing had changed. We knew that his life had just taken a huge step forward and we were soon stuffing our face with the lovely cake The Hearing House put on in celebration.

Now the work really began, and we had a change of therapist from Alexandra to Estelle. She shared this same addiction to silly games as Alexandra but by this stage, I had been beaten into submission, gotten over my manliness and succumbed to their ways. I began to realize that this was all to keep Ollie's interest and that the language and listening were the most important parts.

This brings me to a bit of a digression. Not wanting to sound sexist but I am pretty much a man's man and like manly things, but I found myself wanting to share my experiences with my friends. I would bring things up about what Ollie and I were doing at therapy but the conversation soon ran pretty short and was steered towards more important stuff like fishing, racing cars and drinking beer. From my observations, it is generally the female who does the lion's share of this sort of work, and I have found a new perspective on the importance and challenges faced with childcare as opposed to the importance and skill involved with drinking beer! I had had to step into this role as a single parent and I couldn't be happier at the experience it gave me.

Our weeks were set out in a pretty uniform pattern. Tuesdays were therapy with Estelle. We would drive to the ferry from our home at Onetangi on the Island, get on board and head to Auckland, catch the train to Greenlane and then a twenty-minute walk to the centre. We would do our therapy with Estelle, then head home. During the week, I would teach Ollie for one and a half hours in the morning, then take him to creche. Ollie would spend time with a teacher aide at creche, my parents would then pick him up at 3.30pm and spend the rest of the afternoon with him, teaching him what we had been shown with Estelle. I would pick Ollie up around 5 and we would head home. This was our daily schedule that went on for the next four years. Weekends were a time for me to have a bit of time to myself. Ollie would spend Friday night and Saturday with my parents. I looked forward to that time. When I look back, I think it was a saving grace for me to have that time to myself, not that I got up to much, sleep mainly, but just a time to not have anyone needing my attention. I think it is really important that parents take care of themselves too when taking on a challenge this big.

The first year of therapy was a big adjustment and a lot of work with not a lot of progress, at least that's the way it seemed. Estelle assured me that Ollie was doing fine and that I needed to be patient. I was just waiting for those first words.

We knew he was understanding stuff but still not saying a lot. I guess it was around twelve months into therapy before we started to see some really good progress. Ollie seemed to have put it all together and the words started to come.

Early in the discussions, we were given the option to have both ears implanted, but we would have to pay the $45,000 for the second implant as, at that time, the New Zealand government only funded one implant. I had discussed this with Ollie's mother, and we had opted to wait until we could see whether the first implant was going to work for Ollie.

It was clear now, though, that the responsibility for finding the money for Ollie's second implant would rest solely on my shoulders. I could only raise half the money as my income had been greatly reduced over the last while. I approached a trust on Waiheke that helps children and explained the situation; they were all for what I was trying to achieve and started the ball rolling with $10,000. I was over the moon with this. I had a few things in mind to raise some money myself. One of them was to set up a regular sausage sizzle outside the local supermarket. I didn't expect to make a lot from this, it was more to be seen and be able to speak with people to get our message across. I got the local paper on board and they did several articles on Ollie and myself as we progressed on our journey. The sausage sizzle did really well, we had people come up to buy a sausage and give us $100 and tell us to keep the change. One of Ollie's friend's parents gave us $5,000 and a three-year-old child from Ollie's creche gave us his $2 pocket money instead of spending it on his treat. The whole experience was very emotional and extremely humbling. Our fundraising culminated in an afternoon at a local vineyard where we had live bands, zumba sessions, pony rides, bouncy castle, train rides, a silent auction and lots of fun for the kids. Our song became 'Let's hear it for the boy' on that day. The afternoon's proceeds hit our target. Ollie had his second operation shortly after and all went well.

The second implant proved to be a bit of an adjustment for Ollie. He didn't like it and would constantly take it off or leave it turned off. It took a couple years until both his ears saw equal use. I realise now that this is common as the second implant sounds strange when it is first mapped. Having them done simultaneously would have made a big difference. I am so glad that the government now funds both ears.

Let's hear it for the Boy
A day of music and entertainment including:
AL REEVE
RAHMAN'S ZUMBA
PAT VALICH AND V12
OTHERWORLD PRODUCTIONS
RADIO REBELDE
with MC BRUCE DAVIS-GOFF
At Wild on Waiheke
82 Onetangi Rd
Food stalls
Licensed venue
(Strictly no BYO)
Silent Auction
Kids Entertainment
Eftpos available
Parking $2 at Isola Estate
FUNDRAISER FOR
OLLIE DAVIES
Enabling a deaf child to speak and listen
ENTRY $10 ADULTS

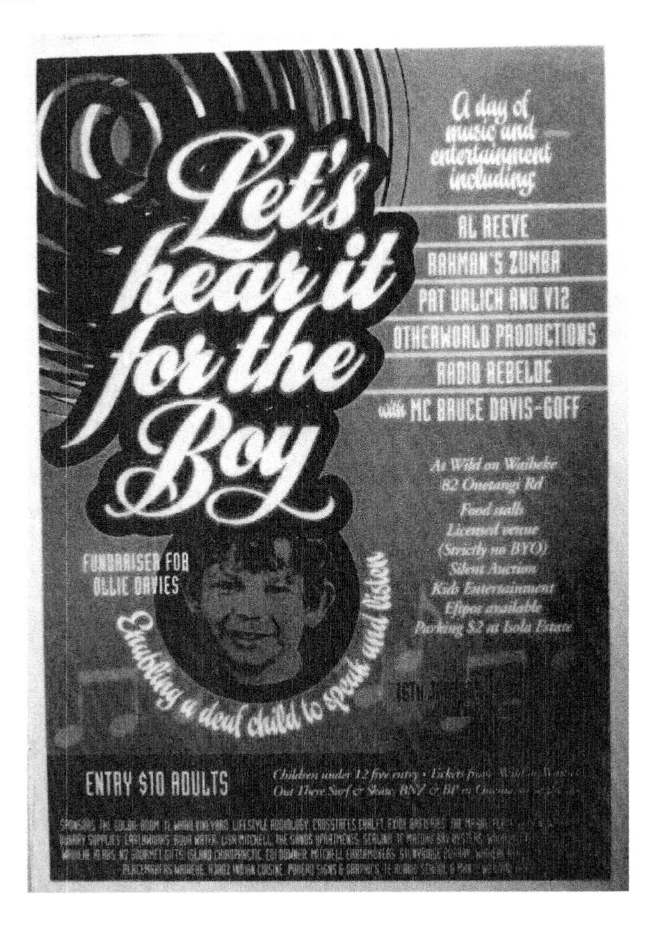

During this time, Ollie and I were involved with the University of Melbourne. Ollie was used as a case study; he was a good candidate as he had one ear implanted two years before the other and we were in a position to give our experience on one versus two ears. The information gathered from us went into a research study looking at the value of two implants which was presented to the government. Shortly after this, the government opted to fund both ears.

Things were progressing well. The Hearing House put together a plus 4 group which consisted of six kids four years and over to help prepare them for school. This was a great thing for Ollie to be a part of as it gave him more interaction in a learning environment with other kids. When I look back, these early years were so important. They set us up for school; there is no way that we would be in a position to attend mainstream school without the help and dedication of our Auditory Verbal therapists, Alexandra, Estelle and Esther, who joined us in our final year.

Starting school was our next step. I would be lying if I said I wasn't a bit nervous about that. My biggest concerns were would Ollie fit in, make friends and cope in an environment with other kids in a mainstream school? I guess many parents feel the same. At this stage Kelston Deaf Education came on board and we were given a resource teacher of the deaf, Catherine, to help Ollie. She would come over once a week and spend the morning with Ollie. We would pick her up from the boat and then drop her and Ollie to school. We got on well and our discussions in the car on the way were really helpful. Catherine also played a big part in Ollie's development. She listened to what we wanted for Ollie which was very important to me.

Ollie started taking swimming lessons at school. These proved to be challenging as he couldn't hear while in the pool. I would come to school and help with him during swimming. I made him take responsibility for his devices, he would put them in a waterproof case and put them in his bag. Being deaf in the pool did not bother him at all. He loved being in the water and would clown around a fair bit. To get his attention, we would donk him on the head with a pool noodle, otherwise he would be quite content goofing off on his own.

We have a trailer boat that we use quite often. Ollie likes being out on the water. One day we called into Garden Cove on the northern side of Waiheke down the 'bottom end'. Ollie and I were swimming around in the shallows. I got back on the boat and saw an eagle ray smooching around not far from us. The ray headed over to Ollie's location and I had no way of letting him know as he was not wearing his devices. I didn't want to frighten him by waving frantically. I was not overly concerned and thought it better to let the ray pass by instead of jumping in as this would likely scare the ray. The ray passed within two feet of Ollie and Ollie was none the wiser. After this incident, we got some aqua covers for Ollie's devices. I can totally recommend them if you spend any time in the water - especially at the beach. They allow Ollie to hear in the water and gave me the peace of mind that I could call to him if I needed to.

One thing we had to deal with was that Ollie would get very frustrated, lash out verbally and throw a big paddy; he really didn't know how to inhibit his emotions and could be very volatile. One day out for a walk at the beach, we were heading home and Ollie didn't want to walk up the hill to our home. He lay down on the road and yelled his lungs out. People were coming out to see what was going on. I left him there and headed up the hill - he soon followed. In our family the road from the beach to our home is now affectionately known as Snotty Road. I spend a fair amount of time with Ollie teaching him to recognise when he is starting to get angry. He was given a card at school that he could show to the teacher when he needed time out - he did not have to give a reason. He would go outside the class or go to the library; this worked really well and he slowly learnt to control himself. I am very proud of him for coping in those situations, as I see plenty of adults who could take a few lessons on the subject.

One thing I was concerned about was that Ollie was spending a lot of time on his own at school during lunch. I used to sneak into the school and watch him out of sight; this was very upsetting for me. We talked about it, but Ollie didn't seem concerned. I think it worried me far more than it did him. I know it is something that many deaf children face and it worries parents but now as a teenager he is able to talk about things that he finds socially difficult and express his emotions really well. It was just another hurdle on our road that was harder for me than it was for him.

One thing that caused a huge change in Ollie was starting to learn guitar. My mother plays and she got him into it; this has been the greatest thing for him. I didn't expect him to persevere with it or do very well but he enjoys it a lot and has kept up with his lessons. We decided to try out doing a bit of busking at the local supermarket, and he got a great response. He has done this three times and it is great to see people stopping to listen and being blown away when they discover that he is profoundly deaf and wears implants. I am very proud of him in this achievement.

In the last twelve months, I have bought him an electric guitar and amp. Initially I was a bit concerned that the noise would be too much for him but he loves it and plays it (at volume) regularly. Last year Ollie did his Grade 5 music exam on acoustic guitar and achieved an excellent result with a 94% pass, something I had never dreamed possible at the start of our challenging journey.

Through The Hearing House, Ollie and I were invited to attend a weekend residence for new parents of children with CIs. We were asked along to be a part of the weekend and for parents to see what progress can be made with kids after a few short years of wearing implants. I gave a talk and shared my experiences with the other parents. One session involved just the dads; that was really great as generally guys don't talk much about these things. In these situations, you find that you are not alone and the issues you face are faced by others as well. I told the group that you need to put your child first and that means PUTTING THEM FIRST, above all else for these first few years. I explained that they needed to step up and help their partner however they could, whether that was hands-on with their child or doing things to lighten the load for the mother. It needed to be their first concern as the best result will come from both of you supporting each other and working as a team. A few years later, I met one of the fathers again and he told me that his family were Cook Islanders and very traditional. The women did the childcare and my talk had made him feel torn between the traditional values placed upon him by his parents and wanting the best for his child. What I had said really hit home for him and he opted to help his wife with all he could and was now so glad that he had a positive role in his daughter's development. Him telling me that was very special.

When I look back, it seems a lifetime ago to the days of despair over being told about Ollie's hearing loss, but I look back with pride in how Ollie has taken things in his stride. Often, I have been the one more concerned than him; he has never complained to me about being deaf. Sure, we have

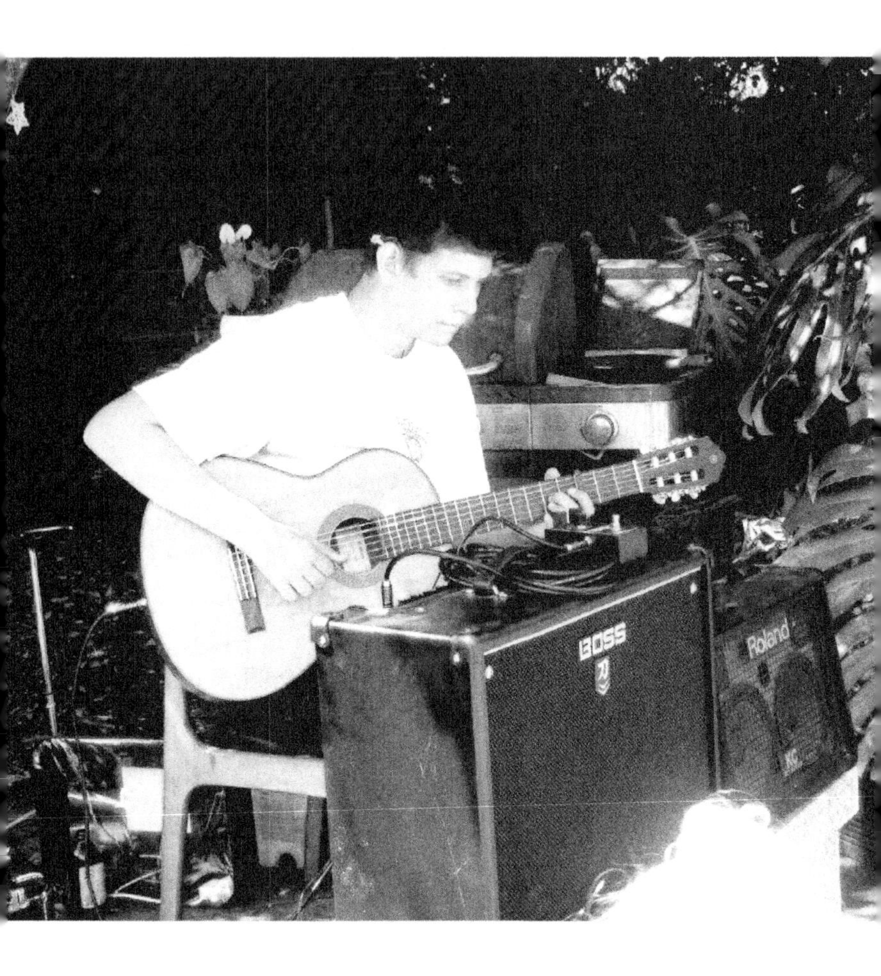
BOSS
Roland

discussed things and the why, but he is, as are most children, resilient and accepting. They just need the love and support from their family. I am a very proud dad and consider myself very lucky that I was the one tasked with steering the ship on the way to Ollie becoming a listening and hearing person who can make his own way in life on the path of his choice.

Having Ollie in my care has definitely changed me and changed my outlook on life. Things that were important just don't seem so important anymore. My parents have always been there for me and my siblings and to a degree I have taken their support for granted. Raising a deaf child as a single working father is challenging but I am extremely fortunate to have had the continued support of my parents for which I will always be thankful. Their input has enabled me to have a balanced life with time for myself, so I did not become bogged down and my time with Ollie was light and happy.

We have not spent much time with signing people, and I genuinely respect a family's choice if they wish their child to sign. We have had mixed experiences with them regarding their views on cochlear implants. Many have been accepting of my decision but there have been incidents when they were clearly against having implants and made their views very clear. One deaf woman who could speak well herself caused a bit of a scene at the sausage sizzle when I was fundraising; she told me that I should be ashamed of myself for doing what I have done to my son. That was a sad experience. I am hopeful that time has calmed these waters and that everyone can respect that a parent has the right to choose.

I do hope your journey will be as positive and enlightening as mine has been.

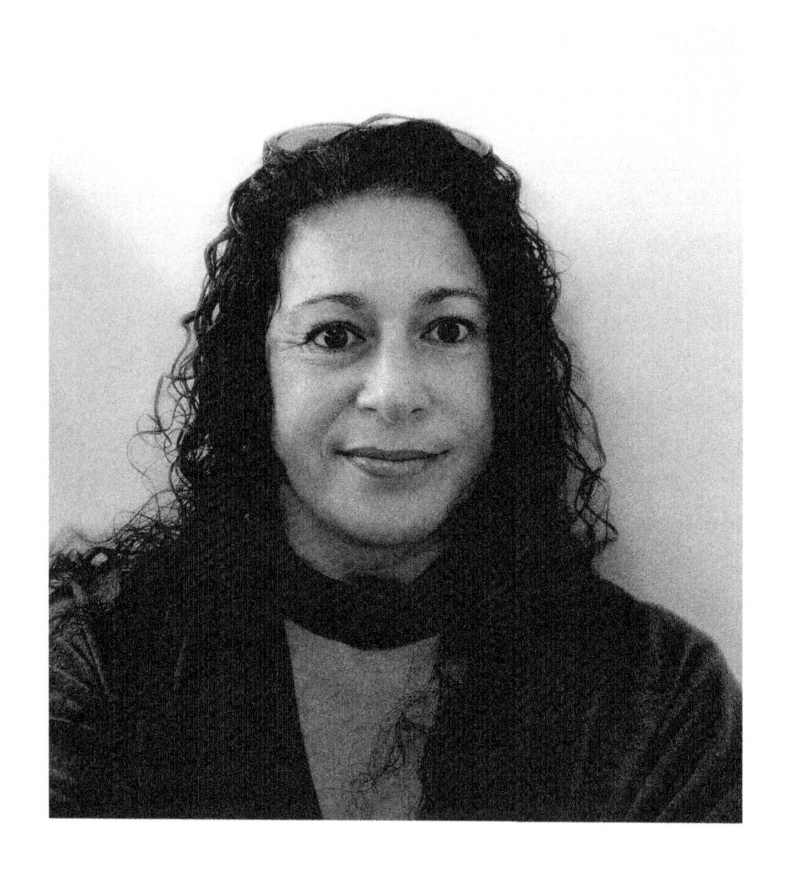

## *Editor's Note*

Throughout my career as an Auditory Verbal therapist, and from my own personal experience too, it has always struck me how it is not just each child's life which is transformed on their journey into the hearing and speaking world, but also that of their families. So many parents and carers have faced new challenges and seen new perspectives on life. They have had to reassess priorities and often start out on completely new career paths to support their deaf children. No one epitomises this better than Esther, an amazing mother who tackled these challenges with fortitude, grace and determination. She tells her own story here, intertwined with that of her children.

**~ Estelle Gerrett**

## Esther and her family's story

# I could do anything with my life, if only...

*I never noticed my ethnicity in the early days but I have definitely noticed the ethnicity thing more as I have become more experienced. I have realised that I do want families/parents like me to know they can do this too.*

My name is Esther and I'm a Niuean-born New Zealander. I grew up in West Auckland, the second youngest of six. Growing up, we mainly associated with my dad's very large Niuean family, as my mother only had one sibling who lived in the South Island.

So, my story started because I wanted a free new phone! Sounds silly, I know, but my sister-in-law had received a free mobile phone by signing up to complete a correspondence course called Mahi Ora (Your Life's Work). I decided to sign up. That was my motivation: a free mobile phone! I can't remember how long the course was - just a few months, but it was a great course. As part of the course, they sent you self-development books to read and one of them was called 'I Could Do Anything If I Only Knew What It Was: How to Discover What You Really Want and How to Get It'. When I read the book it really made me think about what things gave me the most pleasure in life. I realized that I really enjoyed sharing information with other people, even if it was just what was on special at the local supermarket. (My mother-in-law was at a rural address and didn't get junk mail.) As I thought about it more, I began to relate it to the fact that at that time, three of my four children had hearing loss so perhaps that might be something I could explore further. Maybe I could help others dealing with this. I had enough first-hand experience after all. I thought about the adviser on deaf children role and how it was about sharing information with families of children with hearing loss.

With no formal school qualifications, I knew whatever I chose to do was going to be a long road. First I needed to get a teaching qualification, then work for two years as a teacher, and then work another two years with children who have hearing loss. Then another course to qualify as a ToD before I could think of an adviser role. All that was going to cost money... money I didn't have!

I knew it was going to be a challenge with four children at home, but I had been inspired by the book. I knew that there were Teach NZ scholarships, possibly with priority for Pacific and Māori. I decided to look at that. Your income had to be under a certain amount. That was no problem - I ticked all the boxes. I knew even this first step was going to take at least four years because it was part-time and I had four kids, three of whom were deaf. I found that I could study via flexible learning through the University of Auckland and in 2005, I started the course.

There was now another hurdle: no computer or internet access. I needed to be able to study at home, not at a library, so I could be there for my children now aged two, four, seven and eleven. It was great that just then The Hearing House were getting rid of desktops! At last, I had access. This was the beginning of an exciting journey putting my parental experience to use in a professional field. I had so very much to learn but it was exciting!

So, how did all this change my own career path? Well, pretty much before I decided to work towards becoming an adviser on deaf children, I didn't have a career path. I left school close to the end of Sixth Form (Year 12). As for university, well, when I was at school that was just something other people did, not me, not my family. I took a typing course at sixteen, then enrolled in a hairdressing course, and worked briefly as an apprentice hairdresser before I had Jasmin at eighteen years old. Her father and I married shortly after my twentieth birthday and Matthew was born the month before I turned twenty-two. Three years later Jacob was born, and Imari followed two years after in 2002. My other short stints of working were as a nail technician, as an assembly line worker making boxes and vegetable sorting. So, this ten-year plan to become an AoDC was it, this was my career path and the AoDC role was my end goal in terms of a career. I still feel the same. This is my fifth year in the role, and I don't have ambitions to change my job; this is the job I wanted and I love it.

My journey had started many years before when our first baby girl, Jasmin, was diagnosed with a hearing loss at two and a half years old. Later I was to find out that her hearing loss was progressive and would end up profound. When Matthew, our second child, was born he was considered at risk of hearing loss due to Jasmin's diagnosis and the fact that my father had hearing loss. So Matty's hearing was checked routinely at around two months, seven months and nine months; there were no issues but by two and a half he was profoundly deaf. He'd had a progressive loss like Jasmin but Matthew's had declined rapidly. It was a real shock when they told me he had a profound loss as I

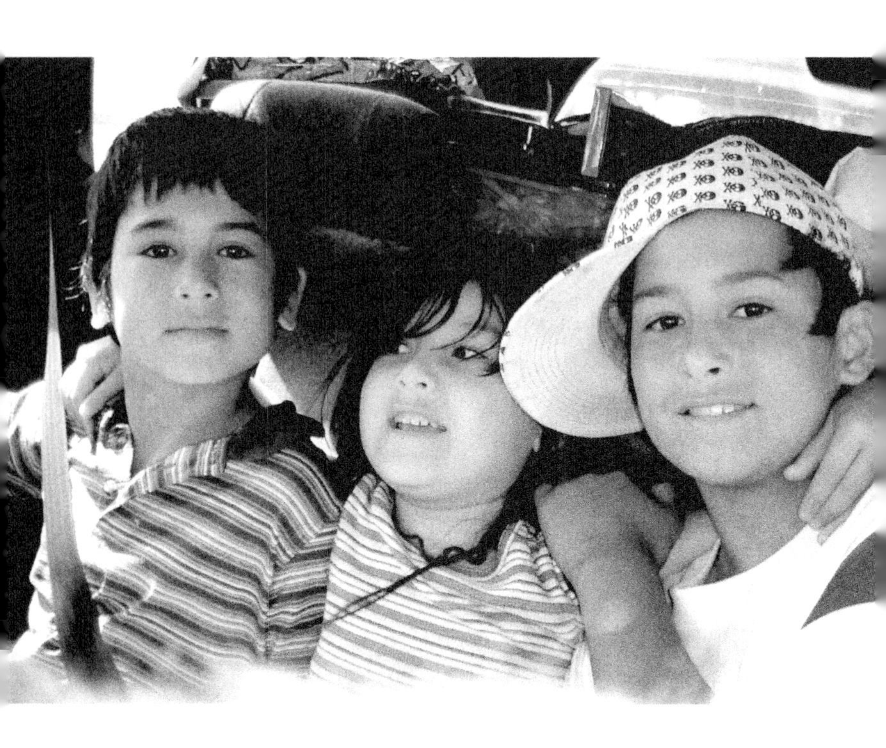

really wasn't expecting that. Even then, I don't think I really realised that it meant he wouldn't be able to speak. He had very little functional language like "No" and "Don't touch". We enrolled Matty in the Kelston Deaf Education Preschool and he and I would be picked up from South Auckland around 7am on a Friday in the preschool van. I remember watching a teacher sign to him at the preschool and thinking he doesn't know what you're saying, he's not used to that. Sign language was foreign for me and foreign for Matty. The people there were so lovely, but we stopped attending as we really wanted him to have a chance of speaking.

I hadn't thought much about deafness affecting his language until I saw an Auditory Verbal therapist, Judy Simser, speak at a local meeting later that year. Part of what inspired me about her story was that she had travelled hours on a train each week to get to the therapy session for her son and then home again. I guess her story hit home because it was this therapy that had supported her to help her son to learn to listen and speak. I decided that this was something I wanted for my son. If she had done it, so could I!

I clearly remember my first visit to The Hearing House and being heavily pregnant with Jacob. Lynne, the therapist who would later work with us, explained to me that it was a big commitment to help a profoundly deaf child to speak. I really took that to heart. I think because I had attended the talk by Judy Simser just before meeting Lynne, I was feeling really inspired and motivated and thought, *I can do this*.

There was still a tough journey ahead for Matty to get a cochlear implant - there were only ten cochlear implants available every year because of funding. Poor Matty, his mother was a bit of snail. I didn't know how to push the system or what I needed to do. I felt I had wasted so much time after Matty's hearing loss was diagnosed. We got heaps of information. I mean heaps! I remember we were given piles of stuff from different organisations and amongst that pile were the documents I'd been given by Matty's audiologist about CI implantation. I just used to put everything in a pile. It was just all too overwhelming! I couldn't face any of it. It was full of jargon and terminology I didn't understand. I've seen other parents do the same since.

I remember the audiologist asking me if I had filled in the cochlear implant documents. I was like, what papers? Thankfully she helped sort it out. We celebrated Matty's fourth birthday. Where had the time gone?!

Matty was such a busy kid. He was a tutū (he had to touch everything and was very good at finding how to get places he wasn't supposed to be!). Just after his hearing loss had been diagnosed, I remember being on the landline phone to somebody and in just that moment, he had climbed out of the window, crawled under the house and gone out the other side. Scary! Little did I know that he had also put a hammer into the tub of our washing machine! I discovered it the next time I did the washing, and the washing machine made a lot of noise! Carer support was offered for Matty and I'm sure it was because when the lady from Taikura Trust came to carry out the interview, Matty was constantly trying to open the back door and climbing into the cupboards, and I had to keep jumping up and down to stop him going out the door. I did worry about his behaviour. He had started getting frustrated with the therapy sessions too before he got his CI. One day, just as we walked into the therapy room, he just swiped everything off the table and started having a tantrum. Lynne (our therapist) was telling him that wasn't okay and he kicked her in the leg. I took him home that day, we didn't stay for therapy. I think this was to do with his frustration at not being understood and what was happening around him. I could have died of shame and embarrassment though.

Matty had his cochlear implant surgery a couple of months after turning four. I felt sound started to have meaning for him quickly, he began to associate the early 'learning to listen' sounds with the corresponding toys quickly, but his language was still so very slow to develop.

Life was very tricky to manage back then. I remember once travelling all the way to Greenlane from Pukekohe on public transport with all four kids for a family fun day, only to find out I'd mixed up the weeks and we were a week late.

I don't remember being really conscious of the fact that I wasn't white, but I was always conscious of feeling like we were somewhere 'flash' when attending The Hearing House – it seemed like a posh kind of place, the kind of place where the people that worked there all looked a certain way. We always dressed nicely to attend. I guess it was seen as a white middle class place. Later I came to understand that these words described what it was that made me feel the way I did; like we were not the same as the people who worked here. It wasn't anything they did, every person we interacted with at The Hearing House was lovely - it was just my self-perception.

One time, the Minister of Health and the Minister of Education were visiting The Hearing House and we'd been asked to attend. It was a big day and I remember realising that one of my sons was wearing second-hand shoes with huge holes in the toes. Oh my gosh, I felt so embarrassed. I can't remember if they were the only ones he had or if I just hadn't noticed that he was wearing them. I'd always been so conscious of our appearances when we went to The Hearing House. I'd always try to make sure we were clean, tidy and dressed nicely.

In 2008, I was in my last year of study toward a Bachelor of Education. That same year Jasmin was in assessment for a cochlear implant, so we still had strong ties with The Hearing House. I was certainly busy enough studying full time with four children and one getting implanted.

The following year there was a vacancy at The Hearing House Preschool and I got the job. I just really loved teaching there. I really loved it. After about six months I was asked if I wanted to train in the therapy clinic. I said, "No, I can't do that, it'll be too hard," but Estelle persuaded me to start just two days a week.

Oh my goodness! When I started, I only had two children on my caseload, but I remember spending hours, like hours, trying to set some short term goals. I'd been asked to set some goals for the little boy on my caseload and I spent ages and ages, still not knowing if I had got it right. It was worse than doing an assignment! I spent so long writing and rewriting the lesson plan, worried I was getting it all wrong. I still remember the first time I was asked to lead an activity in a session... it still makes my eyes water... it wasn't even a session, it was just the Ling Six Sound Test activity and of course we recorded it. Later after I watched it, I went home and I cried and I cried. I cried because I looked so unconfident, so nervous and like I didn't know what I was doing. I felt so vulnerable. After seeing that video, I said to myself I never want to look like that again. Seeing it really made me cry. For the rest of that year I worked two days at the clinic and three days in the preschool and the following year I did three days in the clinic and two in the preschool. My skills were developing.

Coming over to The Hearing House as a therapist was a very big learning journey for me. There were things that I knew which I had learnt as a parent but somehow, they didn't have the same meaning now. When I learned the theory, I got it in a way that I never got it as a parent. Because I had been a parent/client before I began working there, I always had this feeling that I wasn't as deserving of the role and position as my colleagues, as though I sneaked in the back door and that one day someone would find me out. My colleagues were kind and reassuring; these feelings did not come from them, they came from within me.

In my role at The Hearing House, I noticed a connection I felt with my Māori and Pacific families. I loved working with all my families, but I believe there's a different connection when you share a cultural heritage. I recall preparing for a child's first Individual Plan meeting with one of the mums I worked with. It made me recall the first IP meeting I had attended for my daughter Jasmin. I arrived at the school for the meeting; apart from the AoDC and my daughter's teacher, I didn't know who the other three or four people were. They sat around the table talking about my daughter, and at the end asked me if I wanted to say anything. I didn't. I didn't know what to say - I was 'just' a mum. I remembered our AV therapist telling me that I was the most important person at the meeting. Recalling these moments from my own experiences made me determined to ensure that this mum I was working with would have a different experience - an experience that acknowledged her as the mother and expert on her child, where she would be in the know about what the meeting was about, where her voice would be heard and what she had to say would be valued.

As I've become older and more experienced, I've become more and more aware of the ethnicity aspect, my cultural identity and how I feel a strong connection with Māori and Pasifika peoples. I've noticed that I really want other mums like me to know that they can do this too - both for their children and maybe for other families too.

After working at The Hearing House for eight years, an opportunity came up for an AoDC role. I got the job but wasn't ready to leave The Hearing House, so I turned it down. It was too big a change too soon. Later that year another position came up closer to my home and I took it.

Taking that AoDC position led me back to studying again because you needed to get a Master of Special Education (Sensory Disabilities/Hearing Impairment). It was part of the job requirements. I do enjoy the concept of study and I always get excited before I start, but then the work kicks in. Don't get me wrong, I love learning but looming deadlines and rushed submissions, chaotic and crazy days and late nights when time is getting down to the wire, and submitting assessments at the last minute are an all too familiar part of my memories of studying.

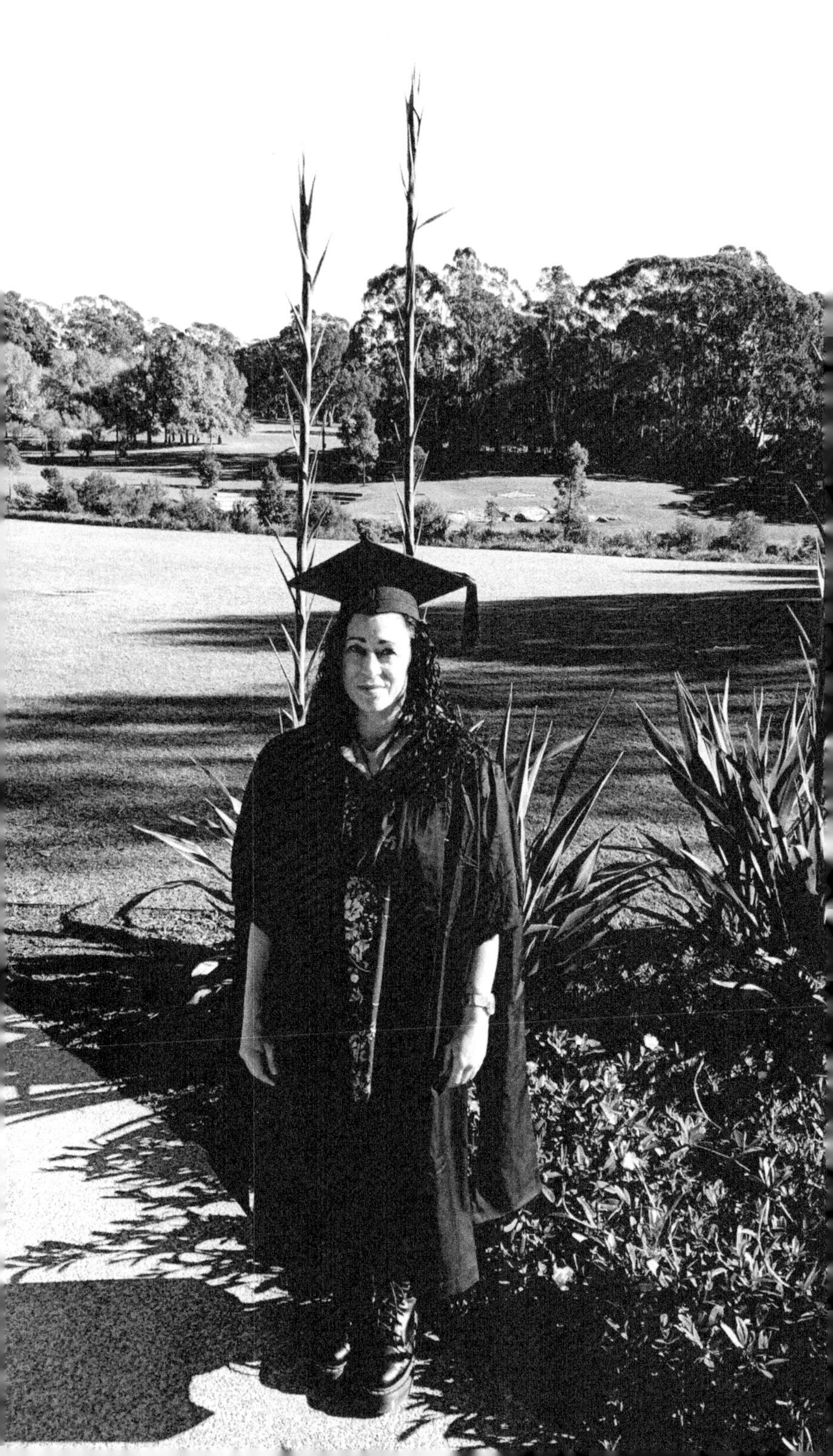

My life has not been a perfect one. My husband and I separated when we were younger, so I experienced life as a single parent raising our four children. I did have great support from family. Years later my husband and I reunited. Jasmin, Matthew and Imari are adults now with their own lives. Jasmin works as a marketing content coordinator, a job she enjoys. Matthew is a father to two children, his eldest daughter has a mild high frequency hearing loss and wears a hearing aid. He recently got his Class Four license and works as a truck driver in a furniture removal company. Imari, our youngest, is renting her own place and works in warehouse dispatch. Our son Jacob was killed in a hit and run incident a few months before his seventeenth birthday. We lost our precious child, our children lost their sibling. In a close family like ours, that was a truly hard and life-changing time. We got through it together but it wasn't easy to navigate.

I love serving the families in our community and I realise there is always more for me to learn. I have spent the last three terms working in South Auckland which has given me lots of opportunities to work with Pacific and Māori families. I am inspired by the families that I work with, families of all cultures and ethnicities, but I do feel an especially strong connection with Māori and Pacific families. There are many roles in the areas of deaf education, where seeing a Māori or Pacific person is not common, but I feel it is so necessary and can make such a difference for the people these professionals are serving.

**I hope you take away from this that no matter where your journey starts, you can make it into what you want, if you fight for it.**

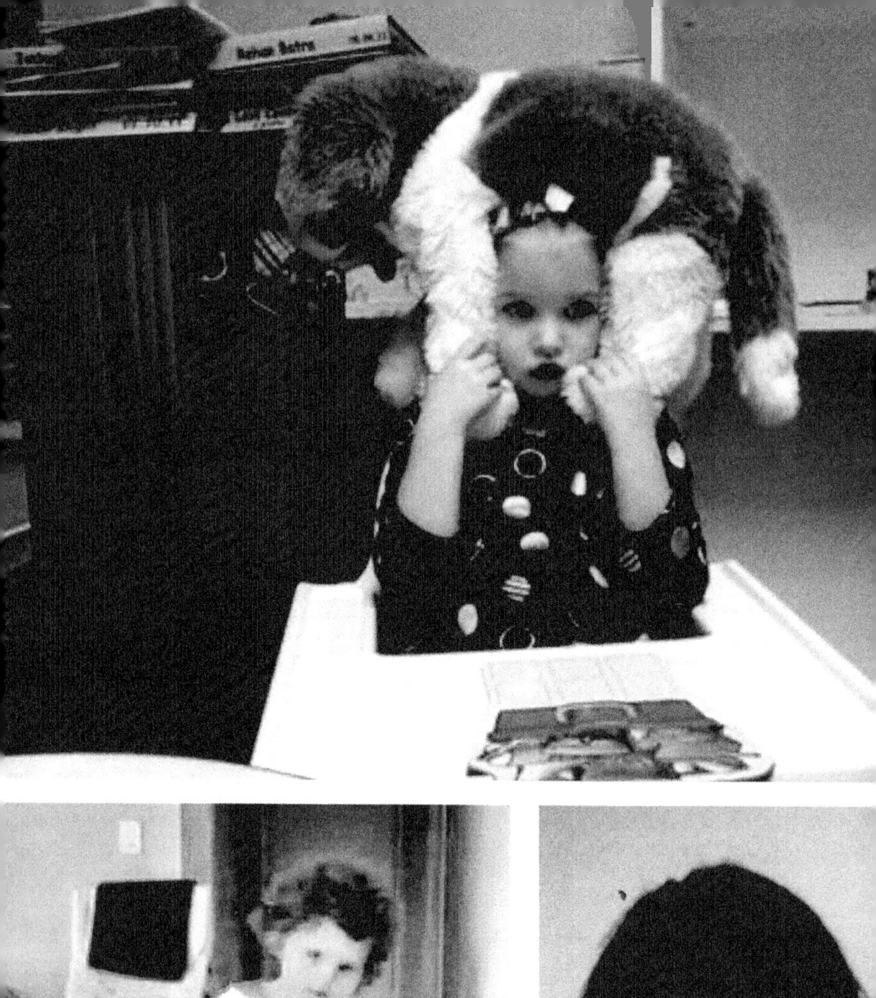

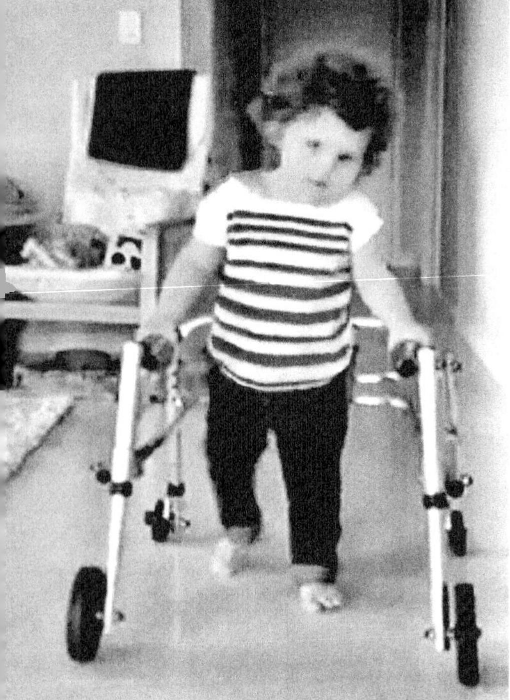

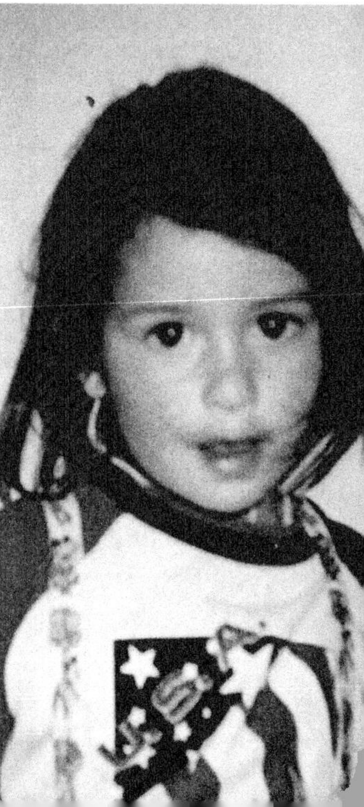

# Acknowledgements

First and foremost, I would like to acknowledge the families who have contributed their stories to this book to help new families find hope in their journey with their deaf and hard of hearing children, alongside all the children and families I have known and worked with over my thirty years in the field. They have taught me so much and I have immense respect for their resilience and determination to give their deaf children every possibility to live a full and rich life.

I would also like to acknowledge the vision and inspiration of the following professionals:
Sir Patrick Eisell Moore and Phil Ryall, founders of The Hearing House, New Zealand;
Annie Ackerman, CEO and driving force of the original Hearing House in New Zealand;
Jacqui Stokes (founder) and Anita Grover (CEO) of Auditory Verbal UK.
It has been due to the management of these inspirational leaders that the families in this book have been able to access Auditory Verbal Therapy.
Lynne Richards, Jacqui Stokes and Liz Fairgray, the clinicians who shaped the clinical pathways and brought the centres to life.
Maree Renee, whose passion inspired me to lift expectations for children with complex needs.
And, of course, the committed surgeons Sir Patrick Eisell Moore, Sir Ron Goodey, Colin Brown and Michel Neeff who changed the landscape of paediatric surgery in NZ.

Without the vision and commitment of these amazing people, the Auditory Verbal vision would never have developed in New Zealand and the UK.

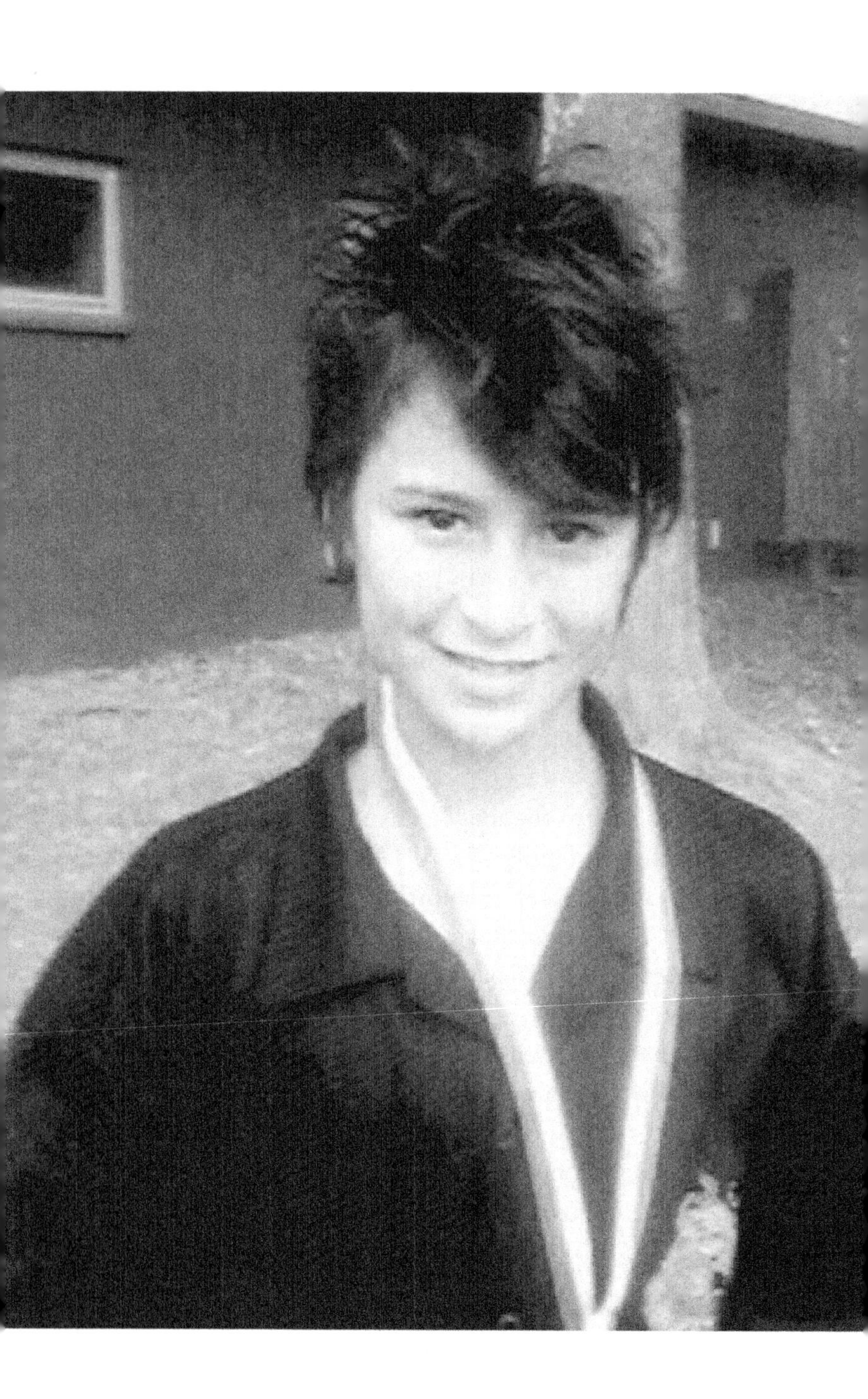

# Notes from the publisher

## Terminology

Because the stories in this book are told by parents in different parts of the world, the terminology they use may sometimes differ from one account to the next. For example, in New Zealand, parents might refer to a "teacher aide" whereas in the UK or USA, this person would be called a "teaching assistant". In other instances, colloquialisms are used, which are particular to the writer's country and not utilised elsewhere. To maintain the authenticity of each account, we have kept each respective writer's original terminology and believe that the context is sufficient to enable the reader to determine the meaning in each case.

## Disclaimer

**Voices of Hope** is an anthology comprising a range of individual personal accounts written by parents of deaf children. The accounts are told in the parents' own words, based on their personal family experiences. Their respective opinions, recommendations and narrative style are entirely their own. The views expressed in this anthology are not necessarily shared by the publisher, AVID Language, or by the collater of the accounts, Estelle Gerrett. We recognise and respect that there are different communication approaches available to families with deaf or hard of hearing children and that each and every family has the right to choose which approach best suits their own situation, diagnosis, culture, values and aspirations.

## AVID Language publishes inclusive books for families with (and without) hearing loss.

We offer books in **English, Spanish & Danish,** with a selection of **British Sign Language** and **American Sign Language** versions free to view on our website.

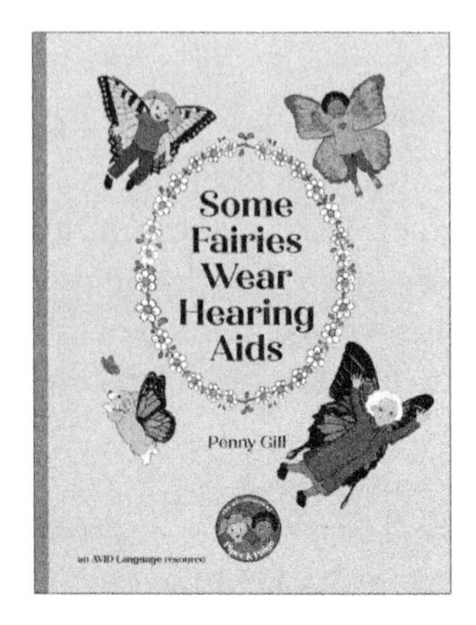


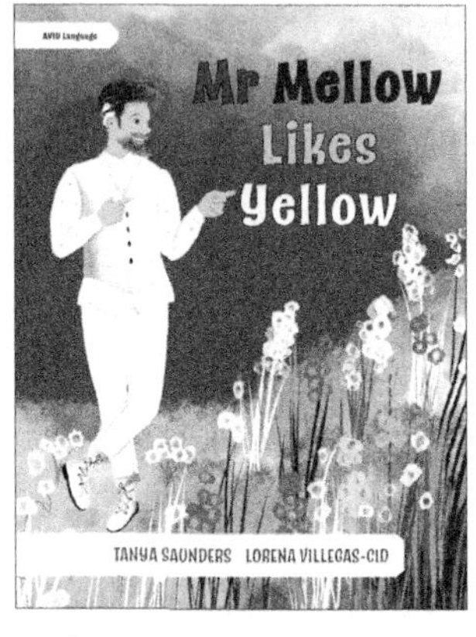


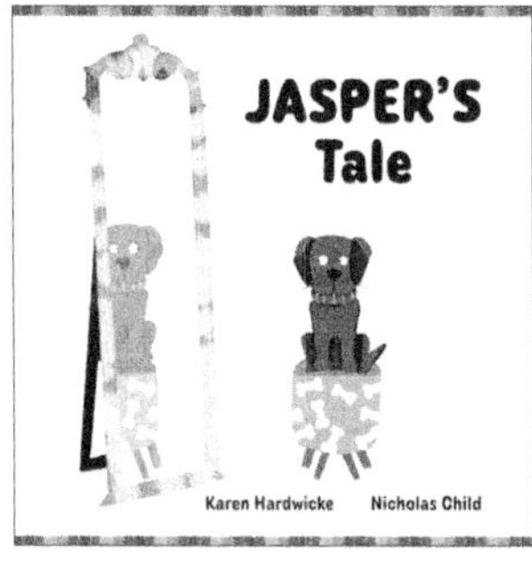


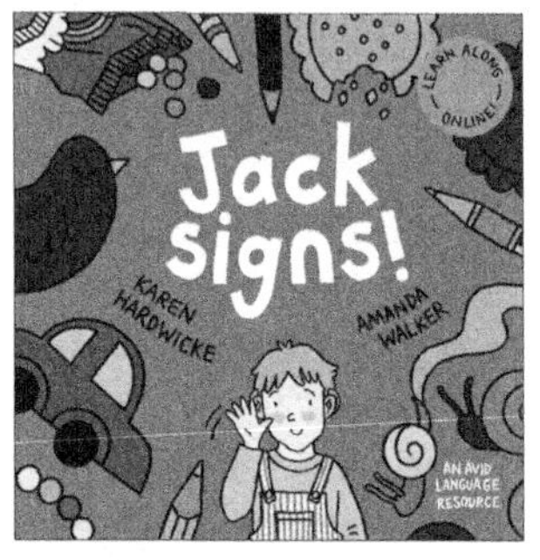


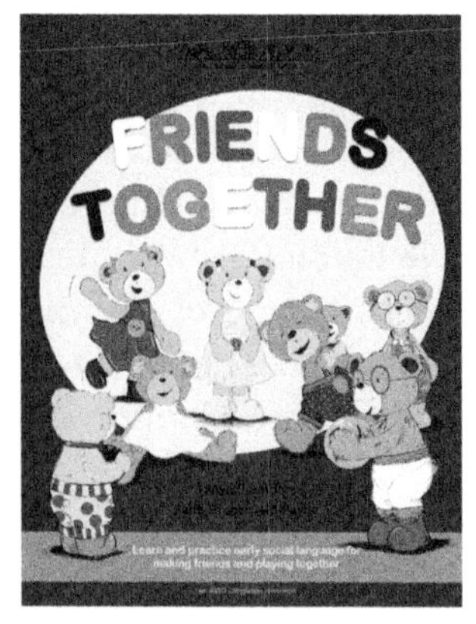


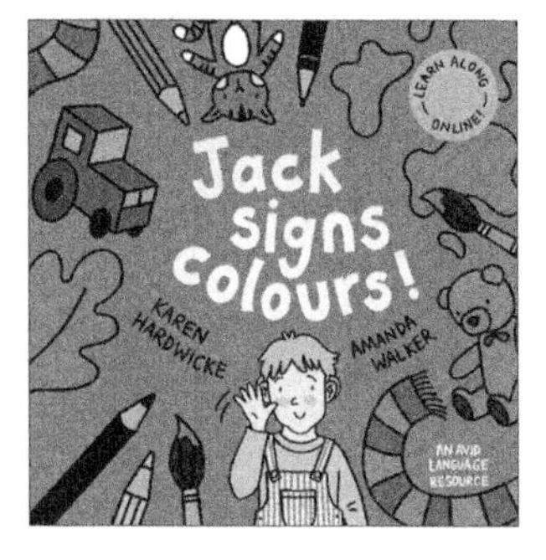

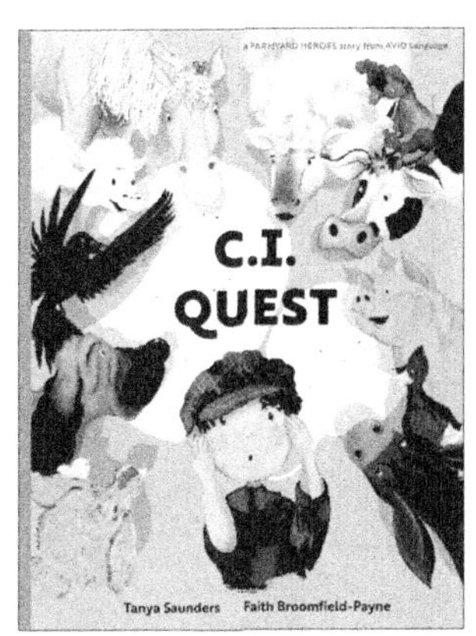


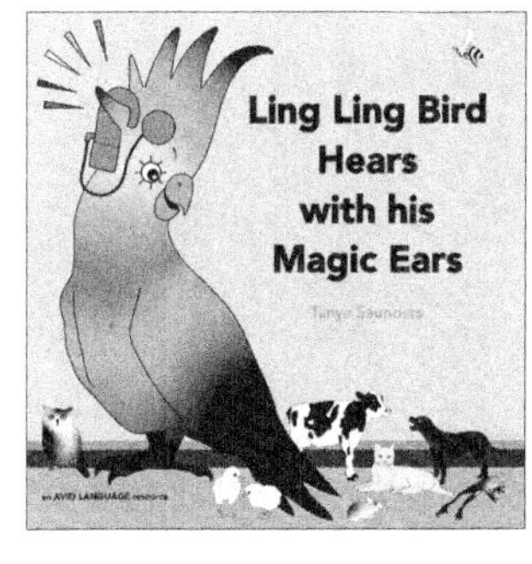


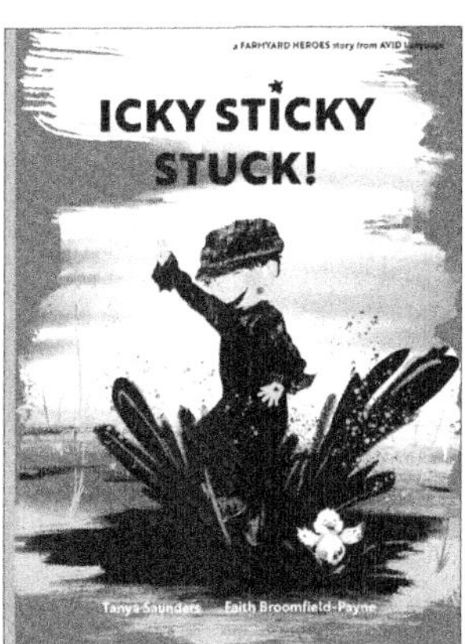


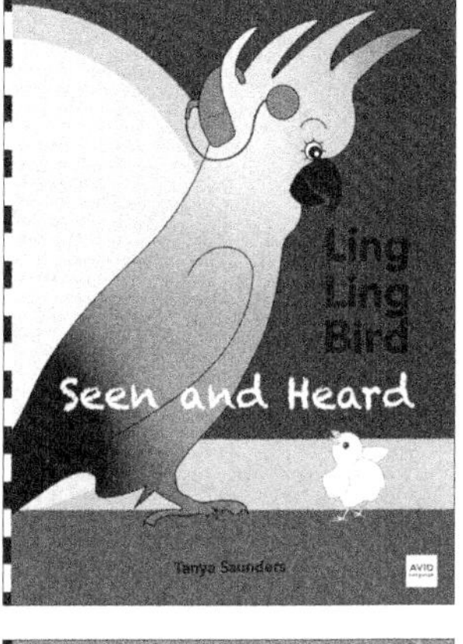


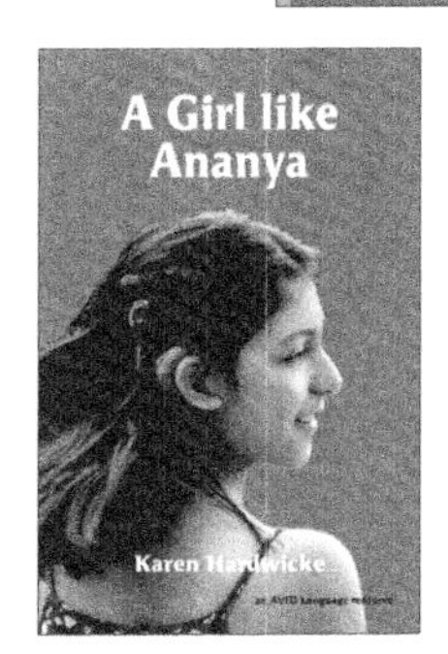


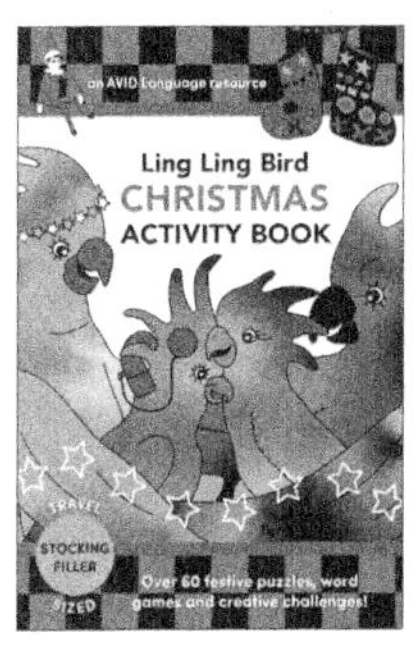


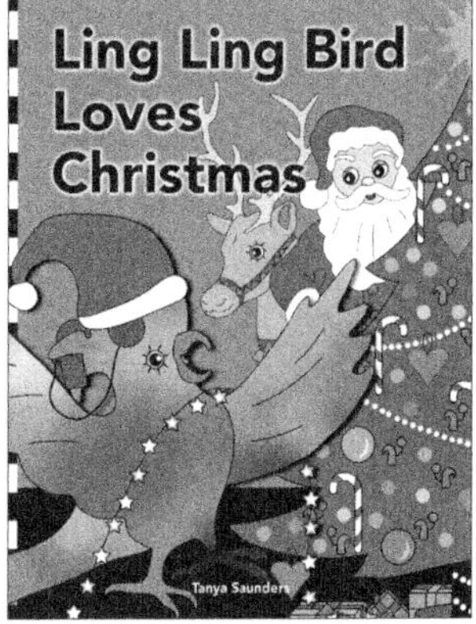


**avidlanguage.com/books**

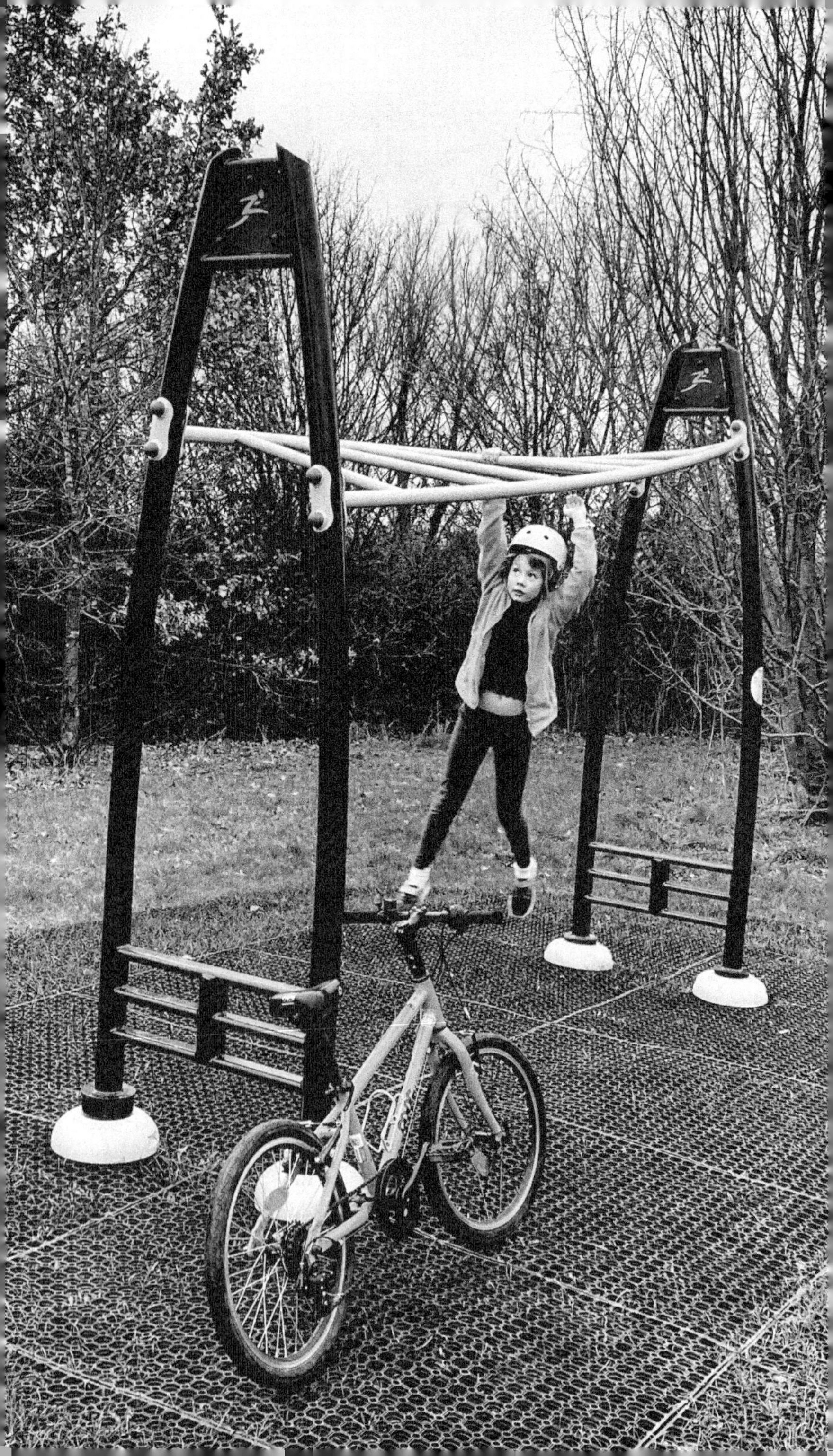

Printed in Great Britain
by Amazon

55227514R00096